HIV/AIDS and Society in South Africa

HIV/AIDS and Society in South Africa

Edited by

Angela Ndinga-Muvumba and Robyn Pharoah

UNIVERSITY OF KwaZulu-Natal Press

Published in 2008 by University of KwaZulu-Natal Press
Private Bag X01
Scottsville 3209
South Africa
E-mail: books@ukzn.ac.za
Website: www.ukznpress.co.za

© Centre for Conflict Resolution
2 Dixton Road
Observatory 7925
Cape Town
South Africa
ccrweb.ccr.uct.ac.za

ISBN: 978-1-86914-152-3

Managing editor: Sally Hines
Editor: Alison Lockhart
Typesetting: Patricia Comrie
Indexer: Ethné Clarke
Diagrams: Marise Bauer
Cover design: M Design

Printed and bound by Interpak Books, Pietermaritzburg

Contents

Acknowledgements

This book is really the result of collaboration between many individuals and institutions. As editors, we have been fortunate to work with some of the most luminous and inspiring scholars and activists in South Africa and beyond. We are indebted to them for their wisdom, tenacity, patience and hard work during the long process of finalising this project.

This volume is part of a wider project initiated by the Centre for Conflict Resolution (CCR), a pan-African, policy-research and training institution, affiliated to the University of Cape Town. CCR would like to thank the funders of its HIV/AIDS and security project: the Rockefeller Brothers Fund (RBF) in New York, as well as the governments of Denmark, Netherlands, Sweden, Norway and Finland, the United Kingdom's Department for International Development (DfID) and TrustAfrica. We want to thank especially Nancy Muirhead and others at RBF, who began supporting CCR's HIV/AIDS and security project in 2004. This volume would not have been possible without their commitment to a long-term research agenda.

We would like to thank Glenn Cowley, Sally Hines and the rest of the staff at the University of KwaZulu-Natal Press, as well as Alison Lockhart, for their generous input, efficiency and commitment to this project. We are also grateful to the skilful and enthusiastic copy editors of the original manuscript: David Le Page, who went through the whole volume, and Ken McGillivray, who helped to complete the process. We would like to acknowledge our colleagues, whose assistance and support ensured the successful completion of this volume: Langa Malimeta, Selma Walters, Elizabeth Myburgh, Dawn Alley, Paul Bradnum, Karin Pretorius and others at CCR, who have helped to plan, organise and administer this project. We are deeply grateful to Adekeye Adebajo, the executive director of CCR, who has never wavered in his commitment to address the HIV/AIDS epidemic in a meaningful way.

Finally, we would like to thank our partners, families and friends, who have given us so much support. These individuals and many others, too numerous to name here, have also been generous with their time and energy, helping to bring this project to fruition.

This book, written on the edge of great sorrow, is but a beginning. We hope it will contribute to an understanding of the way in which HIV/AIDS intersects with political, social, cultural and economic life in South Africa and perhaps offer some answers to those of us who want to change the course of the epidemic.

Angela Ndinga-Muvumba and Robyn Pharoah

Durban and Cape Town, South Africa, 2008

Abbreviations

ACCORD	African Centre for the Constructive Resolution of Disputes
ADEA	Association for the Development of Education in Africa
AEO	Agricultural Employers' Organisation (South Africa)
AIDS	Acquired Immune Deficiency Syndrome
ALP	AIDS Law Project (South Africa)
ANC	African National Congress (South Africa)
APLA	Azanian People's Liberation Army (South Africa)
ARV	antiretroviral
ASCI	AIDS, Security and Conflict Initiative
ASF	African Standby Force
ATM	AIDS, tuberculosis and malaria
AU	African Union
AZT	Azidothymidine (Zidovudine)
BBC	British Broadcasting Corporation
CADRE	Centre for AIDS Research (South Africa)
CBO	community-based organisation
CCETSA	Canon Collins Educational Trust for Southern Africa
CCR	Centre for Conflict Resolution (South Africa)
CDC	Centre for Disease Control and Prevention (United States)
CGE	Commission on Gender Equity (South Africa)
CI	confidence interval
CIA	Central Intelligence Agency (United States)
CINDI	Children in Distress Network (South Africa)
COSATU	Congress of South African Trade Unions
CPS	Centre for Policy Studies (South Africa)
CSIR	Council for Scientific and Industrial Research (South Africa)
CSIS	Centre for Strategic and International Studies (United States)

CSO	civil society organisation
CSSR	Centre for Social Science Research (South Africa)
CSVR	Centre for the Study of Violence and Reconciliation (South Africa)
DCS	Department of Correctional Services (South Africa)
DfID	Department for International Development (United Kingdom)
DHS	demographic and health survey
DNA	deoxyribonucleic acid
DoD	Department of Defence (South Africa)
DoH	Department of Health (South Africa)
DRC	Democratic Republic of the Congo
DVA	*Domestic Violence Act 116 of 1998* (South Africa)
ECOMOG	Economic Community of West Africa's Ceasefire Monitoring Group
ECOWAS	Economic Community of West African States
EDF	Ethiopian Defence Forces
ELRC	Education Labour Relations Council (South Africa)
FAO	Food and Agricultural Organisation
FAO-SAFR	Food and Agricultural Organisation – Subregional Office for Southern and East Africa
FEWER	Forum on Early Warning and Early Response
G8	Group of Eight
GAVI	Global Alliance for Vaccines and Immunisation
GCWA	Global Coalition on Women and AIDS
GDP	gross domestic product
GFATM	Global Fund to Fight AIDS, Tuberculosis and Malaria
GROOTS	Grassroots Organisations Together in Sisterhood (Kenya)
HAART	highly active antiretroviral treatment
HEARD	Health Economics and HIV/AIDS Research Division (South Africa)
HIV	human immunodeficiency virus
HRC	Human Rights Commission (South Africa)
HSRC	Human Sciences Research Council (South Africa)
ICAD	Interagency Coalition on AIDS and Development (Canada)
ICRC	International Federation of Red Cross and Red Crescent Societies
ICRW	International Centre for Research on Women
IDASA	Institute for Democracy in South Africa

IDU	injecting drug use
IFP	Inkatha Freedom Party (South Africa)
IFPRI	International Food Policy Research Institute
ILO	International Labour Organisation
IMF	International Monetary Fund
IOM	International Organisation for Migration
IRRD	Integrated Rural and Regional Development
ISS	Institute for Security Studies (South Africa)
JCIE	Japan Centre for International Exchange
JCSMF	Joint Civil Society Monitoring Forum (South Africa)
KZN	KwaZulu-Natal (South Africa)
MAP	Men as Partners (South Africa)
MAP	Millennium AIDS Programme (World Bank)
MDGs	Millennium Development Goals
MK	Umkhonto weSizwe (South Africa)
MRC	Medical Research Council (South Africa)
MSF	Médecins sans Frontières
MTCT	mother-to-child transmission (of HIV)
NACOSA	National AIDS Convention of South Africa
NAMDA	National Medical and Dental Association (South Africa)
NAPTOSA	National Professional Teachers' Organisation of South Africa
NATU	National Teachers' Union (South Africa)
NGO	non-governmental organisation
NIAID	National Institute of Allergy and Infectious Diseases (United States)
NIH	National Institute of Health (United States)
NPKF	National Peacekeeping Force (South Africa)
NVF	new variant famine
OECD	Organisation for Economic Co-operation and Development
OHCHR	Office of the High Commissioner for Human Rights
OI	opportunistic infection
OVC	orphans and vulnerable children
OXFAM	Oxford Committee for Famine Relief
PEP	post-exposure prophylaxis
PEPFAR	Presidential Emergency Plan for AIDS Relief (United States)
PHC	provincial HIV/AIDS co-ordinator (South Africa)

PLAAS	Programme for Land and Agrarian Studies (South Africa)
PLWA	people living with AIDS
PLWHA	people living with HIV/AIDS
PMTCT	prevention of mother-to-child transmission (of HIV)
POMU	Positive Men United (South Africa)
POWA	People Opposing Women Abuse (South Africa)
PRSP	poverty reduction strategy papers
RAU	Rand Afrikaans University (now University of Johannesburg)
RBF	Rockefeller Brothers Fund (United States)
RHRU	Reproductive Health and HIV Research Unit (South Africa)
RNA	ribonucleic acid
SADC	Southern African Development Community
SADC FANR	Southern African Development Community – Food Agriculture and Natural Resources
SADF	South African Defence Force (now SANDF)
SADTU	South African Democratic Teachers' Union
SALSS	South African Project for Statistics on Living Standards and Development Surveys
SAMHS	South African Military Health Services
SAMP	Southern African Migration Project
SANDF	South African National Defence Force
SAOU	Suid-Afrikaanse Onderwyserunie (South African Teachers' Union)
SAPA	South African Press Association
SAPS	South African Police Services
SARPN	Southern African Regional Poverty Network
SIDA	Swedish International Development Agency
STI	sexually transmitted infection
SWAPOL	Swazis for Positive Living
TAC	Treatment Action Campaign (South Africa)
TB	tuberculosis
TBVC	Transkei, Bophuthatswana, Venda and Ciskei (former homelands of South Africa)
TRC	Truth and Reconciliation Commission (South Africa)
UN	United Nations
UNAIDS	Joint United Nations Programme on HIV/AIDS

UNCHGA	United Nations Commission on HIV/AIDS and Governance in Africa
UNDESA	United Nations Department of Economic and Social Affairs
UNDP	United Nations Development Programme
UNESCO	United Nations Educational, Scientific and Cultural Organisation
UNGASS	United Nations General Assembly Special Session (on HIV/AIDS)
UNICEF	United Nations (International) Children's (Emergency) Fund
UNPBSO	United Nations Peace Building Support Office
UNSC	United Nations Security Council
US	United States of America
USAID	United States Agency for International Development
VAC	Vulnerability Assessment Committee (SADC FANR)
VCT	voluntary counselling and testing
WHO	World Health Organisation
WTO	World Trade Organisation

Introduction

————————— • —————————

Angela Ndinga-Muvumba

*An epidemic that kills young adults in droves spawns difficult politics.
How does a society absorb the death of its young?* (Steinberg 2008, 6)

*Treating HIV/AIDS as any other public health challenge will have to be
accompanied by public commitments by all leaders [in the] political,
religious and private sector[s] to stand by those affected and fight
stigmatisation. The alternative is a downward spiral in our already high
mortality rate and a further reduction in life expectancy.* (Ramphele 2008,
242)

Against the backdrop of the politics of HIV/AIDS in South Africa, a maelstrom of
research and policy development has been produced by and for those who work
with HIV/AIDS every day. However, for those unfamiliar with the literature, how the
epidemic intersects with politics, society and the economy is less vividly portrayed.
Yet, it is a social disease that is shaped by and, in turn, influences South African
society. Where did it begin, and what types of responses are needed to tackle the
epidemic at its roots? How are societal norms that govern our expectations of justice
and equality interacting with HIV/AIDS? What is the disease's impact on those who
lead and protect us? Answers to these questions are complex, sometimes contradictory
and always far-reaching, and knowledge about the intersection between HIV/AIDS
and society emerges through multiple voices, disciplines and practices.

This book is about the ideas that influence how we assess the broader implications
of the HIV/AIDS crisis in South Africa and explores the concept of 'human security'

1

and the global development agenda, both of which emanate from the international political environment and correspond to a discourse on AIDS and society. This volume is also a multidisciplinary overview of the literature. The notion of 'human security' has helped the editors to identify examples of specific areas: human rights, prisons and the military for political security; rural livelihoods, land and development for economic, environmental and food security; and education and orphans for community security. These are imperfect choices and other examples of the intersection between AIDS and society abound in the literature. The police, the mining sector, the health sector, crime and sex work would all be equally useful in such a study. Nevertheless, the contributions in this volume have been selected because they hold relevance for other issues and attempt to answer the questions posed above.

South Africa and HIV/AIDS

South Africa is the prodigal son of nations. With the end of apartheid and its first democratic elections in 1994, the country became, for many, the hope of the world. At the inauguration of Nelson Mandela as president of South Africa in May 1994, Archbishop Desmond Tutu, the Nobel Laureate, was moved to predict: 'Once we have got it right, South Africa will be the paradigm for the rest of the world' (cited in Sparks 2003, 3). HIV/AIDS has tainted this hope and the tragic deaths of millions of South Africans unsettle even the most optimistic observer. According to a national HIV survey, 5.54 million South Africans were living with HIV in 2005, representing 18.8 per cent of all South African adults between the ages of 15 and 49 (South African National AIDS Council 2007a). South Africa's death registration data show a staggering increase in deaths by 150 per cent among women between the ages of 20 and 49 (cited in UNAIDS and WHO 2004).[1]

This book is not about the politics of AIDS in South Africa. There are other books dealing with the African National Congress (ANC) and President Thabo Mbeki's leadership on HIV/AIDS, but it is important to set the scene and to remind ourselves of the political context. The ANC placed the HIV/AIDS crisis on its agenda before it came to power in 1994, but it is widely acknowledged that because of a number of factors, including Thabo Mbeki's leadership on HIV/AIDS, the government has failed to implement an effective policy to deal with the crisis (see Cameron 2005; Gevisser 2007, Chapter 41; Nattrass 2007; Ndinga-Muvumba and Mottiar 2007). AIDS activist groups such as the Treatment Action Campaign (TAC) have been antagonists, friendly critics and partners of the government, playing a pivotal, and at times, controversial role in South Africa's response to HIV/AIDS. Debates about the role of tradition, culture, gender equality, Western medicine, poverty and lifestyle have driven the country's epidemic in numerous directions. For many, this discourse has muted a coherent and frank exchange about sexuality and HIV. Nevertheless, in August 2003, the Department of Health (DoH) initiated the roll-out of antiretroviral (ARV) therapy in public hospitals across South Africa. This was to be guided by an operational plan for comprehensive HIV and AIDS care (DoH 2003).

However, treatment only became widely available in April 2004. ARV delivery to those who needed it most has been described as 'painfully slow' (Hodson 2006). A weak service-delivery structure at the local level is one reason for this. However, the DoH has seemingly privileged prevention over other components of a comprehensive response. This has arguably exacerbated stigma associated with ARV therapy. According to 2004 statistics, KwaZulu-Natal – the province with the highest HIV/AIDS prevalence in the country – failed to meet its treatment goal of treating 20 000 patients by March 2005, and was only treating 3 247 adults and 167 children by the end of 2004 (Gedy, James and Lebea 2004). Yet, by October 2006, 224 895 patients were enrolled in ARV programmes in South Africa (South African Government 2007a), which seemed to indicate that the ARV roll-out was gaining momentum. By the end of 2007, out of an estimated 889 000 people who needed ARV treatment, approximately 488 739 were enrolled in treatment programmes and 371 731 had started ARV therapy regimens (South African Government 2007b, 29).

In April 2007, the South African government put forward a new national strategic plan for HIV/AIDS, which, among other things, proposed to 'reduce the impact of HIV and AIDS on individuals, families, communities and society by expanding access to appropriate treatment, care and support to 80 per cent of all HIV positive people and their families by 2011' (South African National AIDS Council 2007b, 10). Deputy-President Phumzile Mlambo-Ngcuka took on the role of government leader on HIV/AIDS issues and met regularly with civil society organisations (CSOs), in order to forge more constructive alliances in response to the disease. The TAC stated that 'the eight-year struggle to end government HIV denialism and confusion has ended' (TAC 2007). New strategies for preventing HIV, such as male circumcision, also emerged (WHO 2006, 2007). The third South African AIDS conference in Durban (5–8 June 2007) had the theme of 'Building Consensus on Prevention, Treatment and Care' and focused on finding solutions to HIV/AIDS, rather than rehashing old debates about the definition of the problem. Then, in August 2007, President Thabo Mbeki dismissed Nosizwe Madlala-Routledge, the much-admired Deputy-Minister of Health who had been pivotal in the new rapprochement with AIDS activists. Despite the political complications throughout 2007, the government seemed more poised to comprehensively address the epidemic, which it characterised strongly as a grave danger to South Africa. Indeed, the ninth draft (out of ten) of the 2007 HIV and AIDS plan noted that:

> AIDS has been cited as *the major cause* of premature deaths, with mortality rates increasing by about 79 per cent in the period 1997–2004, with a much higher increase in women than in men. Children are a particularly vulnerable group with high rates of mother-to-child-transmission as well as the impacts of ill-health and death of parents, with AIDS contributing about 50 per cent to the problem of orphans in the country. Household level impacts are the most devastating effects of HIV and AIDS in the country. Increases in maternal and childhood mortality are some of the devastating impacts, threatening the country's ability to realise the MDG [Millennium Development Goals] targets of 2015. (South African National AIDS Council 2007b, 10; emphasis added)

Throughout the period after the end of apartheid, an analysis of how HIV/AIDS interacted with society was consigned to the inner sanctum of scholars, or to sound-bites in the media. Evidence-informed research distinguishing HIV/AIDS as a causal factor for the deepening of poverty or insecurity proved difficult to produce. The public debate on how HIV/AIDS affected the country's human resources, for example, was often cast in apocalyptic dimensions.

Human security, AIDS and society

While this book focuses on bringing together different analyses of the intersection between AIDS and society, it is premised on many ideas. One is the concept of 'human security', which encompasses economic, food, health, environmental, personal, community and political security (UNDP 1994). Several contributors use this concept to assess how HIV/AIDS is increasingly being addressed as a security issue, as it facilitates identifying points of entry for assessing the societal implications of HIV/AIDS.

The term 'human security' was first used in a 1994 United Nations Development Programme (UNDP) report, which drew attention to individuals as the fundamental focus of security. Human security was meant to bring to the fore non-military and recurrent security concerns, such as poverty, and to emphasise long-term threats to the life and dignity of individuals, the primary concerns of research on the impact of HIV/AIDS on society (CCR 2006b). In this book, we draw on the broader – and more contested – definition of human security, which includes non-violent threats, such as widespread diseases, environmental degradation, poverty, social exclusion and inequality (Human Security Centre and the Liu Institute for Global Issues 2005, viii; Mack 2004). Human security is also more than a simple, all-inclusive term and focuses on the quality of security for individuals through its emphasis on dignity. Barry Buzan has identified five major factors relating to state security: the military, the political, the economic, the societal and the environmental (1991, 66). This description of security appears to be akin to the notion of human security, and although the contributors to this volume hold diverse views on this topic, they agree on the need to address the epidemic in a holistic way.

As Nana Poku and Bjorg Sandkjaer discuss in Chapter 1, the securitisation of HIV/AIDS has occurred during a time of major transformations in international relations. As a result of the end of the cold war in 1989 and accelerated globalisation, new ideas have influenced traditional notions of security. Human security is an expression that now addresses the outcomes of globalisation and the vulnerability of citizens to insecurity. The HIV/AIDS epidemic poses a great threat to security, particularly in Africa, where seemingly preventable and manageable diseases, such as HIV/AIDS, are prevalent.

Human security also widens the state's agenda and places emphasis on the promotion of human rights, enhanced political participation, access to livelihoods and work and the delivery of social services, such as healthcare and education. Since 1994, a slew of international policy instruments and reports have defined HIV/AIDS as the responsibility of states within this framework. In 2000, for example, the US National Intelligence Council categorised AIDS as a global infectious disease with non-traditional security implications. The United Nations (UN) Security Council under the US presidency held a special session on HIV/AIDS as a security issue in January 2000. In 2004, Kofi Annan, then UN Secretary-General, convened a High-Level Panel on Threats, Challenges and Change, which defined health as an issue of collective peace and security. The Panel's report cited HIV/AIDS as an example of a socio-economic threat to security (UN 2004, 2005).

Moreover, human security and HIV/AIDS have resonated most strongly with development actors. Originating from UNDP, a development agency, human security has come to be equated with development. Combating the disease is one of the Millennium Development Goals (MDGs), which were adopted in 2000 by the UN General Assembly. Based on these policy steps, the expectation arose that the epidemic would be handled by governments and those within the development and security fields in an unparalleled manner.

Alan Whiteside assesses the HIV/AIDS and development agenda in Chapter 10 of this volume. He discusses how development is defined nationally and internationally and examines the relationship between the development goal of reducing child mortality and HIV/AIDS. The year 2005 – 'the year of Africa' – was a year of global commitments made through the United Kingdom's Africa Commission and the Group of Eight (G8) industrialised countries' Gleneagles Summit for Africa's development. However, few of the world's governments grasped how HIV/AIDS could result in greater underdevelopment.

The securitisation of a health crisis also presents conceptual problems. The narrative of security has been written through the language of war: AIDS is the 'enemy', which needs to be 'battled'. The use of war language has helped to mobilise political will, but it has also led to some of the apocalyptic or alarmist images of 'hollowed-out' militaries or failed states. It may have even increased, rather than decreased, AIDS stigma. Furthermore, there is no evidence that HIV/AIDS is a causal factor of state failure or that it fundamentally weakens defence structures (Barnett and Prins 2006; De Waal 2006).

Since HIV/AIDS has a social dimension, evolving within and because of society, it cannot be properly addressed through simplistic classification of the virus as an 'enemy'. Governments cannot go to war with HIV/AIDS without defining enemies within their societies. Instead, they must seek to stop HIV transmission through people's agency and lived choices – an arena far too complex for labels. Pieter Fourie addresses this issue in Chapter 11 and looks at the ways in which AIDS has been securitised at the international level and focuses on the UN's role in shaping the new discourse on HIV/AIDS and security. He also reflects on some of the issues raised by Poku and Sandkjaer in Chapter 1.

The impact of inequality, the weakness of health systems and social, traditional and cultural norms all influence the spread of the virus. For the South African military, these factors also affect the organisational response. In Chapter 9, Angela

Ndinga-Muvumba examines the South African National Defence Force's (SANDF) response to HIV/AIDS. The SANDF has announced that the HIV/AIDS epidemic poses a threat to its capabilities and ability to carry out its security mandate (SAMHS 2005, 2). Given that within sub-Saharan Africa, only a few countries have shown declines in HIV prevalence, commentators have cautioned that Africa's security sector must be urgently protected against the proliferation of the disease. South Africa's military has a 23 per cent HIV-infection rate, which could adversely affect future peacekeeping deployments and the desire to play a leadership role in Africa (SAMHS 2005, 1). The problem of HIV/AIDS – with its demands for labour-intensive palliative care and a lifetime provision of ARVs – also requires management of the defence sector's human and financial resources in a radically different way. Ndinga-Muvumba argues that the defence and offensive capacity of the military are not isolated, but part of a wider spectrum of state functions and responsibilities.

Since South Africa's epidemic is generalised, this book does not focus on target populations – those sectors of society, such as sex workers, which have been identified as vectors of HIV in some societies. Instead it concentrates, for example, on the vulnerability induced by HIV/AIDS through livelihoods or weakened public-sector institutions. Given the level of speculation about the impact of HIV/AIDS, it seems important to illustrate the utility of evidence-informed research to assess who is most vulnerable to HIV within a specific sector and what this portends for the future. In this volume, for example, Chapter 5 examines the status of HIV/AIDS in the public education sector, while Chapters 8 and 9 focus on its impact in prisons and the military – which have been identified elsewhere as having greater levels of HIV prevalence than the general population – and interrogate the response to the epidemic within these sectors.

Roots, rights and vulnerabilities

> *It is a striking fact that wealthy societies riven by social inequality have poorer health indices than societies in which comparable levels of wealth are more evenly distributed.* (Farmer 2005, 20)

Exacerbated by globalisation, the legacy of apartheid's structural inequality is reflected in contemporary South Africa's informal settlements and affluent suburbs. It is also revealed in employment statistics: 35 per cent of South African adults work in the informal sector, but this sector makes up only 7 per cent of the entire economy. Approximately 75 per cent of South Africans have no legal capital to access credit and loans (Sparks 2003, 338–40). Many experts have wondered why HIV/AIDS should be so prevalent in South Africa, which has seen enviable records of economic growth since the 1990s. The sad reality is that wealth has not trickled down (Adedeji 2007) and those people who are the most impoverished are uniquely vulnerable to HIV. Gender inequality and vulnerability to HIV also intersect with poverty in South Africa. For this reason, understanding the roots of economic inequality and its impact on South African society sheds light on the HIV/AIDS epidemic.

In Chapter 2, Shula Marks's succinct social history of HIV/AIDS in South Africa examines how apartheid's expansion of the migrant labour system created a volatile 'high-risk situation', which fuelled the epidemic. The insecurity of life at the apex of apartheid was conditioned by structural poverty, alienation and authoritarianism, which drove policies that cemented inequality and conflict. Based on the multi-disciplinary literature on HIV/AIDS, Marks's chapter illustrates how forced relocations to 'Bantu homelands', the so-called 'mineral revolution' and attendant rapid urbanisation disenfranchised the majority of South Africans. This economic system permanently transformed black family life, sexual practices and the construction of gender identities: the hard life in informal settlements, mining hostels and neglected rural areas depended on the disempowerment of women and the exploitation of men.

It is therefore not surprising that apartheid South Africa nurtured sexual violence and the spread of disease. Troublingly, these patterns have not altered in the last fourteen years and correspond to the HIV/AIDS epidemic's disproportionate impact on women and girls. For every ten HIV-infected men in sub-Saharan Africa, there are on average thirteen women living with the virus (UNAIDS and WHO 2007, 4, 21). In 2005, South Africa's Human Sciences Research Council (HSRC) noted that HIV prevalence peaks at 33.3 per cent among South African women between the ages of 25 and 29, while prevalence typically peaks for men in their thirties and then only at about 23.3 per cent (HSRC 2005, 25). Gender is indisputably one of the most significant factors in determining how HIV is transmitted. Moreover, the confluence of poverty and gender has feminised HIV/AIDS. Women are poorer, on average, than their male counterparts. Social expectations, which govern relations between men and women, continue to underpin the vulnerability of girls and young women to

HIV. While Marks does not claim that the HIV/AIDS epidemic could have been prevented, she does argue that it could be contained. Her chapter leads one to conclude that an effective response must untangle the cultural, social, political and economic circumstances that influence sexual practices in South Africa, and go beyond prevention and treatment of the disease to demolishing structures of inequality and ending the war on women's bodies.

As a result of the HIV/AIDS epidemic in South Africa, health has become a major human rights issue. In Chapter 3, Edwin Cameron and Marlise Richter examine this development within the context of human security. They assess the 'right of access to treatment' and its enforcement, while examining the TAC's legal action against the government in 2002 to provide prevention of mother-to-child transmission (PMTCT) in the form of ARVs through the public health system (see *Treatment Action Campaign and Others v Minister of Health and Others* 2002 (4) SA BCLR 356 (T) and *Minister of Health and Others v Treatment Action Campaign and Others* (No. 2) 2002 (5) SA 721 at 765 at para. 135 E–H). Certainly a progressive rights-based movement in a democratic South Africa is not surprising. AIDS activism – spearheaded by the TAC and other non-governmental organisations (NGOs), such as the AIDS Law Project (ALP), have forged alliances across a wide array of sectors, including religious institutions and trade unions, such as the Congress of South African Trade Unions (COSATU), and kindled what some observers have called 'a second liberation struggle'. The TAC's impact on raising public awareness and legal actions in pursuit of expanding treatment and care through the public health system has strongly influenced current thinking about social change and contemporary South Africa's human rights discourse.

While Cameron and Richter examine the legal implications of HIV/AIDS as a human rights issue, Dean Peacock, Thokozile Budaza and Alan Greig focus on the TAC's grassroots community activists in Chapter 4. They argue that the TAC has been engaged in gender activism of a new kind. Despite the fact that gender-based violence has been widely linked to the rapid spread of the HIV/AIDS epidemic, government and civil society responses have been slow to engineer social change and fuel a revolutionary shift in gender identities. Post-1994 politics have seen a focus on increasing women's participation in the democratic state, but have not led to palpable social change. The TAC's membership, however, is approximately 70 per cent women and the organisation is having an increasingly visible impact on gender issues.

Impacts and responses

Tony Barnett argues that HIV/AIDS is a long-wave event. The epidemic has three consecutive waves or curves: the first is prevalence, the second is AIDS cases and deaths and the third is societal impact (Barnett 2006, 299). It is not yet clear what the societal impact will be 150 years, or even 20 years from now. In many ways, social scientists, policy-makers and politicians are back in 1981, aware that there is a pandemic, but incapable of accurately forecasting just how it will evolve.

A number of analogies illustrate the dynamic of impact between the pandemic and society (CCR 2006a). The more useful of these point out that just as HIV weakens the immune system, the pandemic has the capacity to undermine the social, economic and political health of societies. Moreover, 15–49-year-olds are the most affected by HIV. In 2006, 71 per cent of all deaths in this age group in South Africa were due to AIDS (South African National AIDS Council 2007a, 43). Essentially, the virus is killing off productive, working-age adults and fundamentally altering the country's demographics. The loss of large numbers of current and future soldiers, farmers, teachers, doctors, nurses and other necessary workers poses unique challenges to countries that desperately need human resources to fuel economic growth, contribute to political transformation and transmit knowledge and expertise to the next generation (Ndinga-Muvumba 2005).

However, the evidence is still emerging. Karl Peltzer's contribution to this volume is an important example of how social scientists are mapping the impact of AIDS on society. Chapter 5 is based on a study conducted by the HSRC at the request of South Africa's Education Labour Relations Council (ELRC) (Shisana et al. 2005). The study assessed HIV prevalence among South African public school educators and student educators, finding that rates of HIV were in fact lower than had been speculated. However, the disease is having a critical toll because it reduces the pool of qualified teachers in key areas and demographics. The study found that educators who taught in South Africa's rural areas (and away from their homes) had higher HIV prevalence than those who remained in urban settings. HIV prevalence among student educators – the future of South Africa's education system – was 8.2 per cent and prevalence in African students (13.2 per cent) was higher than that of coloured, Indian or white students combined (less than 1 per cent). Peltzer makes the case for new interventions that target the most vulnerable populations, such as students and teachers in rural areas, in order to prevent future human resource deficits in South Africa's education sector.

An HIV-related illness or AIDS death portends deeper impoverishment for the average South African household. In this way, remaining HIV-negative is also an economic issue. In South Africa, the toll of the disease on livelihoods interacts with issues of access to land and holds particular implications for the livelihoods of people living in communal areas and on commercial farms. In 2004, about 5.3 per cent of respondents to the HSRC survey on HIV prevalence were heads of households where one member of the household was diagnosed as HIV-positive (HSRC 2005, 35). Studies in South Africa and Lesotho have shown how changes in household structure resulting from the interaction of migration and HIV-related morbidity and mortality have weakened people's rights to land. Specifically, the insecure land rights that women typically have make them vulnerable to dispossession on the death of spouses and partners. For southern African countries in which rural poverty is deeply entrenched, this underscores the need to secure land rights, support land-based livelihoods and factor in the challenges faced by those infected and affected by HIV into labour policies. In Chapter 6, Ruth Hall reviews the links between HIV/AIDS and poor rural households. She argues that much of the recent research in this area requires deeper analysis and that too many existing policies are based on national aggregated or qualitative case studies that depict the situation at the macro- and micro-levels, but cannot draw an accurate picture of the way social dynamics, such as land rights, impact on rural livelihoods and, in turn, influence responses to the epidemic in rural communities. On the question of land rights, Hall argues that there have been some adaptations. For example, some cultural practices in parts of southern Africa have evolved to allow women to inherit land. However, these new adaptations are not captured in the policy discourse about human security.

An increasing, but long-delayed concern for policy-makers is the vulnerability of prison populations in South Africa to HIV/AIDS. While public health officials have spent the past 25 years addressing the vulnerability of the general population, prisoners have often remained marginalised. South Africa has a high prison population (160 712 in 2007) and the Department of Correctional Services (DCS) is operating largely overcrowded facilities. In this mix, HIV/AIDS is producing deadly results. The Judicial Inspectorate of Prisons reports that natural deaths in correctional services have increased five-fold between 1996 and 2006, from 1.68 deaths per 1 000 offenders to 9.2 deaths per 1 000 a year (Office of the Inspecting Judge 2007). In Chapter 8, Razaan Bailey focuses on how destructive gender relations among members of prison populations in South Africa create a 'revolving door' of sexual violence between society and prisons, thus exacerbating vulnerability to HIV. Bailey concludes that policy-makers need to adopt a new public health paradigm in the context of prisons and recommends that they should implement harm-reduction strategies, augmenting the DCS's new treatment initiatives, in order to reduce the risk of HIV infection among prison populations.

The HSRC's 2004 survey indicates that there are more than 2.5 million orphaned children in South Africa (HSRC 2005, 35). More than a million children lost one or both parents in 2006 and 69 per cent of the parents who died were the victims of AIDS (South African National AIDS Council 2007a, 43). For some time now, some analysts have linked orphans to increased levels of crime and have been concerned that the epidemic's growing numbers of orphans present a threat to individual and community security. In Chapter 7, Robyn Pharoah challenges assumptions about children orphaned by AIDS, while deepening the analyses of the harsh realities that vulnerable children face. She contends that the causal link between orphans and crime in South Africa is tenuous. Evidence suggests that orphans are more likely to be withdrawn and alienated and that if they are given adequate social protection and support, they are unlikely to turn to crime and violence. Pharoah concludes with a reference to UN strategies for implementing the human rights principles of the *Convention on the Rights of the Child* and promotes this normative framework for action in order to alleviate the suffering of and engender social justice for children affected by HIV/AIDS (OHCHR 1989).

Concluding thoughts

During the last few terrible decades, AIDS has caused the deaths of approximately 25 million people worldwide, or 0.41 per cent of the global population (UNAIDS 2006). However, Africa has borne the greatest HIV/AIDS burden and continues to report higher HIV prevalence, more cases of HIV-related illnesses and greater numbers of AIDS-related deaths than all other regions of the world combined. The 2.1 million AIDS-related deaths in sub-Saharan Africa in 2007 represented 72 per cent of the world's recorded AIDS deaths (UNAIDS and WHO 2007, 47). Southern Africa has become the epicentre of the global epidemic. In 2007, the region accounted for 32 per cent of all new HIV infections and AIDS deaths worldwide (UNAIDS and WHO 2007, 8).

With the arrival of ARV therapy in 1996, the HIV/AIDS terrain was altered permanently. Affordable access to ARVs means that people living with the disease need not die early as a result of the disease, but can live longer, high-quality lives. However, this presents additional challenges. Lifetime provision of universal HIV medication requires human and financial resources, infrastructure development in the health, education and social sectors, as well as political leadership. How will governments that are barely coping with HIV/AIDS establish the conditions that will help them succeed in their struggle against the epidemic? Two-thirds of African countries are spending below 10 per cent of their national budgets on the health sector, while the continent relies on external funding to meet 80 per cent of its HIV/AIDS requirements (African Union Commission 2007, 5). The first 25 years of the pandemic were focused on short-term medical solutions. Given the enormous burden of AIDS on families, communities and states, the next 25 years need to focus on identifying long-term strategies for addressing the human and financial costs of HIV/AIDS on development and democratisation in Africa. There is no better place to begin than in South Africa and this book offers a modest contribution to these efforts.

Note

1. As this manuscript was going to print, it was announced that a study by the Development Bank of South Africa estimated that more than 7.6 million South Africans were HIV-positive in 2007. This is over 2 million more people living with the disease than the number estimated by the South African government (Momberg 2008).

References

Adedeji, Adebayo. 2007. 'South Africa and Africa's Political Economy: Looking Inside from the Outside'. In *South Africa in Africa: The Post-Apartheid Decade*, ed. Adebayo Adedeji, Adekeye Adebajo and Chris Landsberg, 40–62. Pietermaritzburg: University of KwaZulu-Natal Press.

African Union Commission. 2007. 'Draft Implementation Plan for Achieving Universal Access to HIV/AIDS, Tuberculosis and Malaria (ATM) Services, 2007–2010'. Prepared by the African Union Commission, Addis Ababa, April. CAMH/MIN/6 (III).

AIDS Foundation of South Africa. n.d. Statistics available at http://www.aids.org.za, accessed 30 May 2006.

Barnett, Tony. 2006. 'A Long-Wave Event: HIV/AIDS, Politics, Governance and "Security" – Sundering the Intergenerational Bond?' *International Affairs* 82(2): 297–313.

Barnett, Tony and Gwyn Prins. 2006. *HIV/AIDS and Security: Fact, Fiction and Evidence*. Geneva and London: UNAIDS and London School of Economics.

Berhe, Tadesse, Hagos Gemechu and Alex de Waal. 2005. 'War and HIV Prevalence: Evidence from Tigray, Ethiopia'. *African Security Review* 14(3): 107-14.

Buzan, Barry. 1991. *People, States and Fear: An Agenda for International Security Studies in the Post-Cold War Era*. Boulder and London: Lynne Rienner.

Cameron, Edwin (with Nathan Geffen). 2005. *Witness to AIDS*. Cape Town: Tafelberg Publishers.

CCR (Centre for Conflict Resolution). 2006a. 'AIDS and Society in South Africa: Building a Community of Practice'. Report published by CCR, available at http://ccrweb.ccr.uct.ac.za, accessed 17 December 2006.

————. 2006b. 'HIV/AIDS and Human Security in South Africa'. Report published by CCR, available at http://ccrweb.ccr.uct.ac.za, accessed 19 June 2006.

Cilliers, Jakkie. 2004. *Human Security in Africa: A Conceptual Framework for Review*. Pretoria: African Human Security Initiative, Institute for Security Studies.

De Waal, Alex. 2006. *AIDS and Power: Why There Is No Political Crisis – Yet*. London and New York: Zed Books; Cape Town: David Philip. In association with the International African Institute and the Royal African Society.

DoH (Department of Health). 2003. 'Operational Plan for Comprehensive HIV and AIDS Care, Management and Treatment for South Africa'. Pretoria: DoH.

Farmer, Paul. 2005. *Pathologies of Power: Health, Human Rights and the New War on the Poor*. Berkeley, Los Angeles and London: University of California Press.

Gedy, Lloyd, Cheri-Ann James and Motlatsi Lebea. 2004. 'Putting the Government's HIV/AIDS Plan to the Test'. *Mail & Guardian* 30 November.

Gevisser, Mark. 2007. *Thabo Mbeki: The Dream Deferred*. Johannesburg: Jonathan Ball Publishers.

Hodson, Ian. 2006. 'Dazed and Confused: The Reality of AIDS Treatment in South Africa'. Available at http://www.opendemocracy.net, accessed 30 May 2006.

HSRC (Human Sciences Research Council). 2005. *South African National HIV Prevalence, HIV Incidence, Behaviour and Communication Survey*. Cape Town: HSRC.

Human Security Centre and the Liu Institute for Global Issues. 2005. *Human Security Report 2005: War and Peace in the 21st Century*. Oxford: Oxford University Press; Vancouver: University of British Columbia.

Mack, Andrew. 2004. *Human Security Report*. Report prepared for Human Security Centre and the Liu Institute for Global Issues. Oxford: Oxford University Press; Vancouver: University of British Columbia.

Marais, Hein. 2005. *Buckling: The Impact of AIDS in South Africa 2005*. Pretoria: Centre for the Study of AIDS, University of Pretoria.

Momberg, Eleanor. 2008. 'Development Bank Releases Shocking Statistics on AIDS in SA'. *The Sunday Independent* 4 May.

Nattrass, Nicoli. 2007. *Mortal Combat: AIDS Denialism and the Struggle for Antiretrovirals in South Africa*. Pietermaritzburg: University of KwaZulu-Natal Press.

Ndinga-Muvumba, Angela. 2005. 'From Health Crisis to Security Threat: HIV/AIDS and Peace in Africa'. *Institute for Global Dialogue* 10(2).

———. 2006. 'Aligning HIV/AIDS and Security: The United Nations and Africa'. In *A Dialogue of the Deaf: Essays on Africa and the United Nations*, ed. Adekeye Adebajo and Helen Scanlon, 183–205. Johannesburg: Jacana.

Ndinga-Muvumba, Angela and Shauna Mottiar. 2007. 'HIV/AIDS and the African Renaissance: South Africa's Achilles Heel?' In *South Africa in Africa: The Post-Apartheid Decade*, ed. Adebayo Adedeji, Adekeye Adebajo and Chris Landsberg. Pietermaritzburg: University of KwaZulu-Natal Press.

Office of the Inspecting Judge. 2007. 'Annual Report 2006/2007'. Tshwane: Judicial Inspectorate of Prisons.

OHCHR (Office of the High Commissioner for Human Rights). 1989. *Convention on the Rights of the Child*. New York: United Nations, 20 November.

Pharoah, Robyn (ed.). 2004. *A Generation at Risk? HIV/AIDS, Vulnerable Children and Security in Southern Africa*. Institute for Security Studies, Monograph 109, December.

Ramphele, Mamphela. 2008. *Laying Ghosts to Rest: Dilemmas of the Transformation in South Africa*. Cape Town: Tafelberg.

SAMHS (South African Military Health Services). 2005. *The Comprehensive Plan for the Holistic Management of HIV and AIDS in the Department of Defence: 2005–2010*. Pretoria, 5 March.

Scheper-Hughes, Nancy. 1992. *Death without Weeping: The Violence of Everyday Life in Brazil*. Berkeley: University of California Press.

Shisana, Olive, Karl Peltzer, Nompumelelo Zungu-Dirwayi and Julia Louw. 2005. *The Health of Our Educators: A Focus on HIV/AIDS in South African Public Schools*. Cape Town: HSRC.

South African Government. 2007a. 'Government's Programme of Action – 2007'. February. Available at: http://www.info.gov.za/aboutgovt/poa/report/social.htm, accessed 22 February 2007.

———. 2007b. 'Progress Report on [the] Declaration of Commitment on HIV and AIDS: Republic of South Africa, January 2006–December 2007'. Prepared for the United Nations General Assembly Special Session on HIV and AIDS (UNGASS). Pretoria.

South African National AIDS Council. 2007a. 'HIV and AIDS and STI Strategic Plan for South Africa 2007–2011'. Draft 9, March. Available at http://www.womensnet.org.za/services/NSP/NSP-2007-2011-Draft9.pdf, accessed 13 June 2007.

———. 2007b. 'HIV and AIDS and STI Strategic Plan for South Africa 2007–2011'. April. Available at http://www.womensnet.org.za/services, accessed 13 June 2007.

Sparks, Allister. 2003. *Beyond the Miracle: Inside the New South Africa*. Johannesburg: Jonathan Ball.

Steinberg, Jonny. 2008. *Three-Letter Plague: A Young Man's Journey through a Great Epidemic*. Johannesburg and Cape Town: Jonathan Ball.

TAC (Treatment Action Campaign). 2007. 'Government Leadership on HIV/AIDS Irrevocably Defeats Denialism! Implement a New Credible Plan with Clear Targets!' Available at http://www.tac.org.za/AIDSDenialismIsDead.html, accessed 22 February 2007.

UN (United Nations). 2004. *A More Secure World: Our Shared Responsibility*. Report of the Secretary-General's High-Level Panel on Threats, Challenges and Change, A/59/565, December.

———. 2005. *In Larger Freedom: Towards Development Security and Human Rights for All*. Report of the UN Secretary-General, A/59/2005, March.

UNAIDS (Joint United Nations Programme on HIV/AIDS). 2006. 'Report on the Global AIDS Epidemic'. May, UNAIDS/06.20E.

UNAIDS and WHO (World Health Organisation). 2004. 'AIDS Epidemic Update'. UNAIDS/04.E.

———. 2006. '25 Years of AIDS'. UNAIDS/06.20E, May.

———. 2007. 'AIDS Epidemic Update, December 2007'. UNAIDS/07.27E/JC1322E.

UN Commission on Human Security. 2003. *Human Security Now*, cited in Japan Centre for International Exchange (JCIE). 2006. *Report on Monitoring and Evaluation Mechanisms for the Projects Supported by the United Nations Trust Fund for Human Security in the Field of Health and HIV/AIDS*. New York: Japan Centre for International Exchange.

UNDP (United Nations Development Programme). 1994. *New Dimensions of Human Security*. Human Development Report. New York: UNDP; Oxford: Oxford University Press.

Uvin, Peter. 1998. *Aiding Violence: The Development Enterprise in Rwanda*. West Hartford: Kumarian Press.

WHO (World Health Organisation). 2006. 'Regional Consultation on Safe Male Circumcision and HIV Prevention'. Report based on the meeting of the UN Regional Working Group on Male Circumcision, Nairobi, Kenya, 20–21 November. Available at http://www.who.int/hiv/topics/malecircumcision/MCregconsultationNov2006.pdf, accessed 1 June 2007.

———. 2007. 'WHO and UNAIDS Announce Recommendations from Expert Consultation on Male Circumcision for HIV Prevention'. Press release, available at http://www.who.int/mediacentre/news/releases/2007/pr10/en/index.html, accessed 23 March 2007.

From State Security to Human Security

—————•—————

Nana Poku and Bjorg Sandkjaer

Introduction

The concept of 'human security' was given its empirical content in the Human Development Report, *New Dimensions of Human Security*, published in 1994 by the United Nations Development Programme (UNDP). The idea has subsequently gained tremendous currency in both policy and academic circles. However, human security has yet to become a robust analytical and policy tool. While the idea has been applied indirectly to a number of issues, ranging from violent to non-violent threats, upon further scrutiny, human security appears to lose coherence.

The gap between human security as a concept and its policy relevance is a paradox. On the one hand, there is debate about the analytical rigour of the concept, since virtually all economic, food, health, environmental, personal, community and political upheavals could conceivably constitute a threat to human security. On the other hand, the broadness and inclusiveness of the term 'human security' has served to elevate, as well as unite political mobilisation for a broad range of policy issues, such as socio-economic rights, thus creating a new paradigm for development. Indeed, human security alternates between being a theoretical concept explaining the state of the world, to being part of the very world that needs explaining.

This chapter is divided into three parts and examines notions of security in a changing, globalising world and explores the observation that HIV/AIDS may threaten security in southern Africa's most HIV-affected countries. The first part deals with the realist conception of security in international relations and traces the emergence and subsequent dominance of realism. The second part addresses what is meant by human security, as this is a relatively new term in international relations literature and diplomatic parlance. We explore the relevance of the human security approach for understanding the outcomes of globalisation and the vulnerability of African citizens to insecurity. The third part of this chapter illustrates how using the concept of human security can expand our understanding of the impact of HIV/AIDS on states and societies, focusing on southern Africa as an example of how the pandemic interacts with governance and economic development.

Security in a changing world
Realism and security

For almost half a century, cold-war ideology served to eclipse the distinction between the state (defined as an internationally recognised government in control of a specified territory) and the multiplicity of values, claims and identities of a state's citizens. In matters of security, state and society were considered one; thereby ignoring what was and is arguably a problematic relationship. In general, states' policies during the cold war appeared both well defined and comprehensive to include everything that mattered to their national interests. Importantly, the national interest denoted the core collective objectives of the state. In descending order of priority, the collective objectives were deemed to comprise the security and survival of the state, economic prosperity, and the sustenance of the social and political values of the security of the state. Veteran US diplomat, George Kennan, offers the clearest elucidation of the cold war's ideology:

> Government is an agent, not a principal. Its primary obligation is to the interests of the national society it represents, not to the moral impulses that individual elements of that society may experience . . . The interests of the national society for which government has to concern itself are basically those of its military security, the integrity of its political life and the well being of its people. These needs have no moral quality. They arise from the very existence of the national state in question and from the status of national sovereignty it enjoys. They are unavoidable necessities of a national existence and therefore not subject to classification as either 'good' or 'bad'. (1985, 206)

Kennan's exposition is indebted to the methodological insights of the dominant international relations theory of the time: realism. Whether situated against the early twentieth-century crisis of historicism, or analysed as yet another benighted footnote to dualism inherited from classical Greek philosophy, claims to political realism in the theory of international relations carry meanings and implications from a broader discourse about politics, philosophy and community. Central, however, is the argument that any serious extension of moral and political community beyond the boundaries of the sovereign state is inconceivable in the context of anarchy. As such, the state becomes the censorious referent of security and the concept becomes synonymous with the defence of the national interest.

Embedded in the realist position are deep assumptions about the basic character of humanity itself: that the struggle for power is inherent, universal and reified in a propensity for violence in the conduct of sovereign states towards each other. Externally, the state has to be strong because it confronts others like itself – hence the conception of the international system of states as anarchic. The result is a decentralised system where conflict is endemic and security is managed by self-help. Each state has to provide for its own security; each must arm itself.

In this realist worldview, socio-economic considerations are subordinate to military considerations. Although states engage in international exchanges, such as trade, this engagement is fragile because they must worry about the relative gains accruing from such exchange, which could directly affect their relative position of strength and power. In the realist worldview, there can be no permanent friendships or enmities, only constantly changing alliances dictated by no other sentiment than the survival of the state.

However, theories are not isolated from the interests and political realities of their time (Gadamer 1983). The genesis of realism lies in the ruins of the Second World War. The lessons learnt by critics of that era's interwar diplomacy led them to the conclusion that the causes of the Second World War were largely the naive legalistic and moralistic assumptions of the liberal idealism characteristic of the interwar period (Carr 1964). The threat of nuclear war further served to consolidate the view that conflicts of interest among states are inevitable and as such, the purpose of statecraft is national survival in a hostile environment. Threats to states' security principally arose from outside their borders and were primarily, if not exclusively, military in nature and often required military responses, if the target state was to be preserved. State sovereignty was therefore a cornerstone of international law, giving heads of states the freedom and – Kennan would argue – the responsibility to do whatever is necessary to advance the state's interest and survival.

The end of the Second World War coincided with the emergence of a unique geopolitical system dominated by two superpowers, the United States and the Soviet Union. The cold-war period was characterised by the stockpiling of nuclear weapons and periodic crises that threatened to erupt into global violence of apocalyptic proportions. Not surprisingly, these crises seemed to confirm the realist emphasis on the inevitability of conflict, the poor prospects for co-operation and the contest of national interests among incorrigibly selfish, power-seeking states.

On both sides of the ideological divide, one state (the United States in the West and the Soviet Union in the East) monopolised political decisions through a mixture of coercion, inducement and, frequently, force. Within each state, the pervasive ideology of the cold war served to fudge the distinction between states and popular interests, or the uneven representation of different categories of people within the security projects of states. The cold war therefore made it possible for analysts to legitimise states' policies with respect to citizens by placing the domestic domain beyond the parameters of inquiry. For the analyst, the referent object of security became the state.

The post-cold-war era, globalisation and security

Today, territorial, ideological and material boundaries are attenuated, unclear and confusing. The post-cold-war world is not simply 'disorderly', but complex: an environment that appears fragmented and polarised, while at the same time, it displays remarkable integrative features (Poku and Graham 2000). There continues to be a widespread recognition of the need to reconceptualise the foundations of the emergent global order. The debate over whether a clash of civilisations is the dominant feature of our times is illustrative of this recognition, as is the burgeoning literature that posits the possible emergence of global civil society (see, for example, Huntington 1996). For many analysts, the transition out of the cold-war ideology has been jarring and requires a reappraisal of the philosophical assumptions from which the realists constructed the cold-war world.

The complexity of the post-cold-war world is heightened by globalisation. The literature on globalisation generally asserts that the phenomenon is a process whereby states are being integrated into a world economy. Roland Robertson notes, however, that globalisation also refers to cultural and subjective matters, namely, the scope and depth of consciousness of the world as a single place (1992). In a manner that is reminiscent of Francis Fukuyama's claims about the 'end of history' (1992), globalisation is also seen as the latest in a series of Enlightenment narratives purporting to outline a universal civilisation and a common destiny for humankind (Albrow 1996). Globalisation has simultaneously been denounced as being a concept of economic reductionism, technological determinism, political cynicism and defeatism (Gills 1997). Yet, even if the meaning of globalisation remains in doubt, the principal agents of the changes rendered in the post-cold-war world are evident enough, such as globalising corporations emerging from a rapid process of super-mergers, techno-scientific networks and the aesthetic architects of mass culture (Dicken 1992). There has also been a shrinking of the world brought about by the so-called 'third technological revolution', which has enabled us to travel both vicariously and instantaneously to almost all regions of the world (Allen and Hamnet 1998).

The process of globalisation, therefore, is tearing away the traditional notion of continuous, historical time, on the one hand, and established spatial parameters, on the other hand. In the process, it is radically altering the manner in which we conduct our lives, in the sense that locales become thoroughly penetrated by and also shaped by social influences quite distant from them (Poku and McGrew 2007). Anthony Giddens argues that such changes are reconstructing social relationships across reorganised time and space (1990). More than any other development, the blurring of the internal-external divide by the forces and processes of globalisation brings into sharp focus the notion of security and insecurity in the modern world. In the words of former US president, Bill Clinton, 'there is no longer a division between what is foreign and what is domestic – the world economy, the world environment, the world AIDS crisis, the world arms race – have all become global in nature and reach' (*The Washington Post*, 21 January 2005).

What these comments perceptively challenge is the conception of two separate worlds, in which domestic security is set against contrasting insecurity outside. In truth, the polarity has always been artificial, but it is rendered even more so under the conditions of globalisation. As such, the binary oppositions that shape our interpretation of violence, between private (criminal) and public (legitimate), or between external (international) and internal (civil), can only be applied with difficulty to the contemporary world (Kaldor 1998). Human security, a concept predicated on the confluence of numerous issues linked to the rights to dignity and to life, has emerged as a new articulation of the merging of boundaries between the poor and rich in a globalising world (for more on the relationship between human rights and human security, see Chapter 3 in this volume).

Human security and Africa

The first decade of the post-cold-war world demonstrates in the most tragic way the exposure of vast numbers of people not only to the dangers of violence from contending bands of warriors and bandits in a manner reminiscent of medieval times, but also to hunger, disease and poverty on a cataclysmic scale. For many people in the most affected societies, the chief security threat is the very government under whose sovereignty they live, either through its oppressive policies, or as a result of its incapacity to sustain the infrastructure of life for the vast majority of its people. Conflicts in the Democratic Republic of the Congo (DRC) and Rwanda in the 1990s and the ongoing conflicts in Sudan and Somalia, for example, underscore the plight of populations without protection from external aggressors and their vulnerability to predatory states that are supposed to be their protectors. Thus normative claims for privileging the state are untenable: to view threats to humanity simply in terms of protection from military violence by other states is problematic in the modern world.

The authors of the 1994 UNDP Human Development Report had this in mind when they coined the term 'human security'. The concept of 'security', the authors of the report argue, has been too limited when restricted to questions of territorial integrity, or threats such as a nuclear holocaust. For the majority of the people in the world, apparently marginal or esoteric concerns – such as environmental security, food and economic security – are far more real and immediate threats to their daily survival than interstate wars. The authors of the report strongly criticise the focus on state security as a way of ignoring the concerns of daily survival for the world's people (UNDP 1994). The UNDP critique argues that security must be viewed in ontological terms and the state as that which can be threatened from a number of directions and by agents and actors who are not necessarily other states.

Nowhere has the expanded notion of security been more applicable than in sub-Saharan Africa. Unlike in Europe, where nation-builders sought to replace the older empires with states founded on some combination of cultural, linguistic and patriotic unity, African states emerged from the authoritarian structures of their colonial past. Any analysis of security and insecurity in contemporary Africa must therefore begin with the 'abnormality' of the African state (for a review of literature on the African state, see, for example, Ake 1996; Bratton and Van de Walle 1997; Clapham 1996; Fatton 1992; Iliffe 1995). With callous disregard for the histories of their subjects, colonial leaders grouped large numbers of diverse identities, ethnicities and cultures into new states, while dividing nations with rich and unified histories into separate states. The partition of the Somali people of the Horn of Africa is a typical example. Previously united by a common culture, but lacking a centralised authority, this classically segmented political system was ultimately subjugated and divided among four imperial powers: Britain, France, Italy and an independent Ethiopia. Regardless of whether one is sympathetic to past or current Somali demands to redraw the inherited colonial boundaries of the Horn of Africa, there is no question that the roots of the conflict in Somalia and elsewhere in Africa are, at least partially, the result of illogically drawn European colonial boundaries (Poku 1996).

Total order, in the Hobbesian sense, therefore has thus been virtually impossible to achieve in Africa. Indeed, the biggest challenge to modern African leaders has been consolidating the nation-states bequeathed to them by colonialism. In some states, the dominant traditional nation became the core of the new nation, as other ethnic groups were assimilated into it or marginalised. Wolof in Senegal, American-Liberian in Liberia, Hutu in Rwanda, Shona in Zimbabwe, Baganda in Uganda and Amhara in Ethiopia were the key elements in defining the new nations as the cultural basis of the new state. In other states, an artificial creation was decreed and all traditional nations were dissolved into it; those who could or would not fit were excluded. President Mobutu Sese Seko of Zaire (named Congo before and after his reign) instilled a Zairean identity among the many ethnic groups of the DRC, which was so strong that it outlived both him and the change of the country's name back to the Congo again (Weiss and Carayannis 2005). Despite the claims to national unity that post-colonial African leaders extolled, the state and its leadership were always alien from the social base on which their power rested. The African state is arguably therefore less a nation-state than anywhere else, despite, or perhaps because of, the efforts to make it so.

If African states are artificial in origin and lack strong legitimacy, how do they keep going? Commitment to the state in Africa has, in many respects, been bolstered by those who benefit from it, expressed through the institutions of government of which they form a part. As long as a state's own hierarchy and the social groups forming it remain intact, it is very difficult for anyone else to challenge it. The collapse of the state, or the mounting of any secessionist movement dedicated to its dismemberment, has invariably been prompted by deep divisions within the governing class or elite: the fragmentation of the Nigerian officer corps under the stress of coups and massacres in 1966; the destruction of the old Ethiopian government and the bloody struggle for succession after the 1974 revolution; the dissolution of the Somali Republic into clan rivalries; the shattering effects of despotic military rule in Uganda in 1972 and the inability at any time to create a unified governing community in states such as Sudan, Chad and Sierra Leone are all cases in point.

States are said to collapse because they are unable to carry out their functions effectively as states (Zartman 2005). One of these key functions is the legitimate monopoly of force. Many states in Africa are not able to claim the legitimate monopoly of force in the Weberian sense, because both the ostensible monopoly and its legitimacy are contested. Hence, there are countries where security is challenged by both rebellion and internal dissent, such as in Senegal, Guinea-Bissau, Liberia, Côte d'Ivoire, Ghana, Nigeria, Chad, Sudan, Ethiopia, Somalia, Kenya, Uganda, Rwanda, Burundi, Congo, Angola and Zimbabwe. In all these states, although the government is accepted, the political institutions through which its powers are exercised are treated with remarkable indifference by large sections of the population. While this passive acceptance might not be as problematic in other contexts (one often hears about the disenfranchised or disenchanted electorate in Western Europe and North America), in the African context, it serves to deepen insecurities by alienating people from the apparatus of the state.

Finally, governing elites in Africa have often had to form compromising alliances to augment their hold on political power. This includes reaching out to militias, such as the Jeunes Patriotes in Côte d'Ivoire; the Kamajors and Civil Defence Forces in Sierra Leone; Ninjas in Congo-Brazzaville; Janjaweed in the Sudan; civil defence forces in Zimbabwe and militias in the DRC, which serve as 'official rebel armies' to enforce partisan security and impose their own will. At times, states have also opted to farm out security to private and public mercenaries at great cost to their own functional legitimacy (Reno 1998; Roberts 2006). Contemporary private mercenary forces include companies such as Executive Outcomes, Sandline International and Military Professional Resources Incorporated. For more legitimate military deployments, African states have been assisted by United Nations (UN) peacekeeping operations, a large number of which are operating in Africa: in January 2007, about 70 per cent of UN peacekeepers were deployed in Western Sahara, Liberia, Côte d'Ivoire, the DRC, Ethiopia/Eritrea and the Sudan (see United Nations Department of Peacekeeping Operations n.d.). The African Union (AU) has deployed a peace operation in Sudan's Darfur region that is now a hybrid UN-AU force. Regional peacekeeping operations, such as the Economic Community of West African States' (ECOWAS) Ceasefire Monitoring Group, intervened in conflicts in Liberia, Sierra Leone and Guinea-Bissau in the 1990s.

Contemporary African states have, evidently, rarely been blessed with the unifying influence of strong, homogenous nationalism. This has given rise to a situation where individuals make greater attachments to their localities (or local communities) than to the overarching state. Indeed, the 'vast majority of Africans now regard their governments as irrelevant or as purveyors of indifference and cruelty' (Cheru 1989, 2). When we take these circumstances in sum, it is little wonder most of the world's so-called 'collapsed states' (Zartman 1997) are in sub-Saharan Africa.

Yet, if we remove territorial boundaries from our cognitive map, we are left with a picture of people across sub-Saharan Africa attempting to pursue security within the hostile environment of weak states. Across the continent, governments preside over fractured societies with a multiplicity of ethnic identities and divergent interests, making it particularly difficult to generate a legitimate basis for governance. Meanwhile, ordinary Africans lurch between an alien superstructure (the state) and a decaying traditional African past. As many head to the melting pots of ever expanding cities, their loyalties stretch between predatory elites and disintegrating tribal systems (Ake 1991, 7).

In the African context, therefore, the notion of security only makes sense if it is conceived in its broadest context. The 2004 Non-Aggression and Common Defence Pact of the AU offers the following definition: '[In Africa] human security means the security of individuals with respect to the satisfaction of the basic needs of life; it also encompasses the creation of the social, political, economic, military, environmental and cultural conditions necessary for the survival, including the protection of fundamental freedoms, access to education, healthcare, and ensuring that each individual has opportunities and choices to fulfill his/her own potential' (African Ministers of Defence 2004). This definition thus embraces issues such as human rights; the right to participate fully in the process of governance; the right to equal development and access to resources and the basic necessities of life; the right to protection against poverty; the right to education and good health conditions; the right to protection against marginalisation on the basis of gender and protection against natural disasters, as well as ecological and environmental degradation. The AU framework embraces the whole gamut of civil, political, economic, social and cultural rights. In the process, it constructs a radical account of politics as freedom from domination and exploitation, as well as material sufficiency.

A word of caution: notwithstanding the obvious synergy between the UNDP definition and the AU's formulation, it would be a mistake to overstate their convergence. While both assert the importance of human security, they differ quite markedly on the role of the state in this process. The UNDP definition questions not only the ability of the state to provide security, but equally importantly, its role in propagating insecurity. The breadth of the UNDP definition proved problematic for the AU, not least because it risks conflating the quite different agendas of international security, on the one hand, and social security and civil liberties, on the other hand. Thus, while the AU readily accepts the case for focusing on the interplay between the international and domestic security agendas, it cautions against a reductionist approach that prioritises individual security above the collective security of the state. For the AU, embracing the notion of human security involves devising a formulation that encompasses both the traditional, state-centric, notion of the survival of the state and its protection by military means from external aggression, as well as the non-military notion, which is informed by the new international environment and the high incidence of intrastate conflict.

It is therefore possible to envisage the AU framework as representing a radical attempt to relocate the security discourse, to move it from the abstract terrain of international relations discourse and to embed it in the socio-political and economic realities of the African continent. In Africa, state security is rarely threatened by conventional armed attacks by other countries, but usually by more insidious influences, many of which arise from the weakness of the African state itself (see Buzan 1991). Without effective national security, neither citizens nor communities can be personally secure in the broader sense of the term. Without secure and stable countries and a body of practice or law – whereby countries regulate their interactions – individual, community, regional and international security remain elusive.

AIDS, security and instability

In the case of most life-threatening epidemics, the onset of disease is quickly followed by serious illness or death. The cumulative effect of deaths due to the Ebola virus, multiple-drug-resistant tuberculosis, or the avian flu can be registered in months. This is not the case with HIV/AIDS. Initial HIV infection is followed by a lengthy period of mostly asymptomatic incubation, lasting in most African cases for five to eight years until illness and death as a result of AIDS. Only once the AIDS stage has spread sufficiently throughout the population does the epidemic start to have a visible demographic impact. Thus, the epidemic has been characterised as slow acting. HIV/AIDS' lengthy evolution also masks the general effects on individuals and their households, which absorb the shock of reduced incomes and increased costs for healthcare. Conceivably, this slow-acting epidemic's cumulative effects over many years also produce significant changes across a society. Assessment and delineation of these changes, however, has proved elusive.

The HIV/AIDS epidemic has resulted in the death of 22 million Africans – most of them aged 15–49, people in their potentially most productive years – with effects that will continue and echo over coming generations (AU and UN 2006). Among southern African countries, the greatest increase in mortality has been registered among adults aged 20–49. While this group accounted for 20 per cent of deaths between 1985 and 1990, by 2006 it comprised 60 per cent of all deaths (UNAIDS 2006, 4). Life expectancy will decline in Botswana, South Africa, Zambia and Zimbabwe to 30–45 years by 2010 (UNAIDS 2006, 81). As a result of these demographic changes, there will be fewer people, especially in the 20–50-year-old age group, to contribute to the management of national affairs, whether in government, business, religious or social life (UNDESA 2005). Some countries already report that increased morbidity and mortality resulting from AIDS exacerbate the existing skills shortage, particularly in sectors such as education and health, but also at all levels of public service.

These worrying demographic changes only indicate the wider reach and impacts of the epidemic. If we assume that for each of the 22 million AIDS deaths during the course of the epidemic, five people within the immediate African family are directly affected, then over 100 million Africans are closely affected by the epidemic (Poku 2005, 60). To the millions already lost to AIDS, those currently battling HIV and their families, must be added those less directly affected in extended families, colleagues at work, close friends in faith groups and other communities. Thus, a staggering proportion of Africa's people are personally affected by HIV/AIDS.

The impact of HIV/AIDS on human security
The first and greatest impact of AIDS deaths is at the level of individuals and households, with the burden of care falling to girls, women and the elderly and a

depletion of productive labour and resources (Whiteside 2002). There are important analyses that examine various coping mechanisms and adaptations, suggesting that there is a great deal of variability in the way the epidemic impacts on families (see, for example, Chapter 6 in this volume). Nevertheless, many households affected by HIV/AIDS must manage the negative impacts of the costs for treating illness and the loss of productivity. A 2002 study shows that in South Africa's Free State province, HIV/AIDS-affected households tended to have monthly incomes one-third less than non-affected households and also that they spent less on food (Booysen and Bachmann 2002). Households manage loss in a number of ways, including seeking wage labour through migrancy, switching to low-maintenance subsistence food crops, liquidating savings, reducing consumption and tapping into the extended family. A 1998 survey reveals that in Zambia, chronically ill heads of households reported reducing the area they cultivated by half (Waller 1998). Namibian studies have revealed that the chronically ill have devoted less attention to livestock, leading to the deaths of their animals (Engh, Stloukal and Du Guerny 2000).

Failing initial coping strategies, households must then sell off land and other assets or begin borrowing. The most destitute households break up and become dependent on charity. In the South African province of KwaZulu-Natal, households where an adult member had died of HIV/AIDS were three times more likely to be dissolved than other households (Hosegood, Herbst and Timaeus 2003, 14). A 2004 study of HIV-affected households in Zimbabwe found that where the adult female head of a household had died of AIDS, 65 per cent of the households were dissolved (UNCHGA 2004, 12). Surviving the impact of AIDS can eventually lead to dire circumstances: increasing use of child labour, removal of children from school, increased demands on the community for cash and gifts, transactional sex and begging. The intuitive link between the impact on households and the public sector is clear. Eventually, resources to assist the most heavily affected households and their communities will have to be provided by the state's health, labour and education sectors (Donahue 1998).

Given the prevalence of HIV in southern Africa, development will require a scaling up of healthcare, basic social services and job-creation. However, the possibility that the pandemic will outpace any accelerated HIV/AIDS response and related development strategies poses an additional concern. Arguably, the aggregate indirect economic impacts of HIV/AIDS could include an increase in poverty and therefore, reductions in tax revenues, while there is an increasing demand for services. Policy-makers can only be certain that the macro-level impact of HIV/AIDS will emerge incrementally in a non-linear pattern (Poku 2005, 118). However, for many of the poorest countries in this region and the rest of Africa, the deferral of development translates into a threat to stability.

As many countries are still in a relatively early stage of the HIV/AIDS epidemic, the long-term political ramifications are unclear, but it is possible that it might act as a destabilising force in many countries. In southern Africa, with increasing immediacy, the epidemic poses the challenge of ensuring that democratic transitions continue, despite the instability caused by HIV prevalence as high as 10–30 per cent of adult populations. As explained above, the loss of human productive capacity, through the disruption of livelihoods, will have the greatest impact on the poorest of the poor, who will constitute an important segment of the disenfranchised. Less clear will be the impact of increased mortality as segments of the general population succumb to AIDS. How this will affect democratic transitions in southern Africa remains a major concern to policy-makers. While the poorest will suffer the greatest loss in terms of their livelihoods, HIV/AIDS will also affect millions of teachers, civil servants and healthcare workers – those at the very frontlines of the response to the epidemic (see, for example, Chapter 5 in this volume on the impact of the epidemic in the public education sector in South Africa).

In South Africa, for example, AIDS was the biggest single cause of death among young adults in 2000 (Bradshaw and Dorrington 2005). Yet, it remains unclear how these AIDS deaths influence political participation and thus the priorities of the state (De Waal 2006). Arguably, the very constituency that would seek to increase social services to combat the epidemic is also the group that is most likely to remain invisible in political processes: the stigma of AIDS, the costs of managing the disease and the disproportionate impact of HIV on young women and their inequality all render this group less likely to be actively engaged in political participation (for more on the ways in which gender relations in South Africa influence HIV prevalence, see Chapters 2, 3 and 4).

That the epidemic is concentrated in areas already undergoing tenuous economic transitions only heightens the risk of instability and insecurity. Until recently, the most common method for projecting the long-term economic effects of HIV/AIDS was to estimate the effects by projecting the impact of the epidemic on gross domestic product (GDP) (see Bonnel 2000). This method has an important shortcoming: it does not fully take into account the reduction in welfare due to the loss of family members.[1] Recent research attempts to address these shortcomings include using a broader definition of welfare that includes the monetary value of the changes in life expectancy, as well as per capita income. Under conservative assumptions, the conclusion is that Africa's mortality changes already imply an economic cost of HIV/AIDS equal to 15 per cent of 2000 GDP. This translates into a decline in income of 1.7 per cent per year from 1990 to 2000 (Bloom, Canning and Jamison 2004), which exceeds previous estimates based solely on the loss of output as a result of the epidemic. In the case of a typical African country with HIV prevalence at 20 per cent, GDP would be 67 per cent less at the end of a twenty-year period. One implication of this is that highly affected countries will sink into greater poverty.

As such, the cost of HIV/AIDS to societies and economies becomes much greater than the figures usually quantified by economists. This derives from the compounding effects of the epidemic on vital human capital, which serve to cripple the capacity of low-income countries to develop an effective response to HIV/AIDS. Because the education and health sectors are vital to the implementation of prevention programmes in schools and providing medical care, the loss of human capital increases the odds that HIV/AIDS epidemics will remain strong and last longer. Over time, declining human capital and lower investment combine to reduce the productivity growth on which long-term per capita income growth depends.

As the human resources and capacity of governments and agencies are lost to HIV/AIDS, the ability of the state to carry out its functions is impaired. Although comprehensive and conclusive evidence on this point is still elusive (Elbe 2003), for the hardest-hit countries in southern Africa, these losses of human capacity are almost certain to leave states less, not more capable of protecting and providing for their citizens. The question for policy-makers and academics trying to assess security in this context is whether or not these weaker states in democratic and development transitions will be able to sustain effective governance, political legitimacy and stability in the years to come.

Securitisation and HIV/AIDS

For some commentators, the securitisation of humanity is quite problematic, not least because it risks mixing up the quite different agendas of international security, on the one hand, and social security and civil liberties, on the other hand. Barry Buzan, for example, questions the analytical validity of human security as a concept and argues that it is a reductionist approach (2004). Roland Paris underscores this argument, noting that definitions of human security are, in the main, imprecise and sprawling, and address vastly different issues from physical security to mental health. This, he argues, provides policy-makers with little guidance in prioritising competing policy demands, and academics with little sense of what is to be assessed or critiqued (2001).

Individuals are not free-standing: they take their meaning from the societies in which they operate. The individual cannot be reduced or subordinated to a single referent outside of the society in which he or she operates. So, if those who have framed the concept of human security have sought to collapse all the possible referent objects for security into a single object, caution is necessary, as this excludes the claims of both collective and non-human referent objects, such as the environment, in a way that defies other moral claims, as well as the actual practices of securitisation. Indeed, reductionism of this type would not only eliminate the distinctiveness of international security – which is focused on interaction among social collectivities – but would also challenge the viability of security studies as a sub-discipline within international relations. Fundamentally, there is a need for greater prioritisation of the issues covered under the umbrella of human security and, related to this, the development of improved analytical tools to better understand these issues.

In reality, it is possible that both Buzan and Paris have missed two central features of the concept of 'human security'. First, although the concept focuses on the inviolability of the individual, the vast majority of literature on human security addresses institutions as the guarantors of human security. Human security policy generally analyses the capacity and responsiveness of states at the domestic level (government services, the judiciary, parliaments and the executive) and at the international level (through institutions such as the UN and the AU). Second, far from being a reductionist concept, human security should be conceived as emancipatory, encompassing and empowering the hopes and aspirations of a group of people – academics, development practitioners, non-governmental organisations (NGOs), community-based organisations (CBOs) and donor organisations – for a better world. This would be a world in which children are not allowed to die from preventable diseases, where epidemics such as HIV/AIDS are not allowed to decimate an entire continent, ethnic prejudice is not allowed to result in gratuitous violence (or worse, genocide), where women are not illegally trafficked or sexually abused and corruption is not allowed to continue to reduce millions of people to a bleak and vulnerable future.

These are issues with an emotional charge of a kind that only a subjectifying narrative can fully convey and around which a coalition of forces are needed to bring about radical political changes (see Chapter 11). Ironically, it is precisely this subjective, emotive and practical facet that has traditionally served to also exclude the discussion of these issues at the appropriate political level.

Conclusions

For fifteen years, government responses to the HIV/AIDS epidemic were ineffective. In January 2001, the most powerful political organ of the UN, the Security Council, held a special session on HIV/AIDS (for more on this, see Chapters 10 and 11). The most interesting observation, at least for our purposes, was the fact that this was the first time that the Security Council had met on an issue not directly related to traditional security issues, such as the threat of armed conflict between states. The headline of *The New York Times* report on the session was: 'UN Redefines Aids as Political Issue and Peril to Poor' (Steinhauer 2001). The important observation about this headline is not the fact that the Security Council's members framed HIV/AIDS as an issue of the right to life or to dignity, nor indeed, that the epidemic affects the poor disproportionately. The critical point is that the Council perceived HIV/AIDS to be an issue with potential implications for global security.

When HIV/AIDS was just another plague of the impoverished and marginalised, to be endured along with malaria, tuberculosis, or manifestations of malnutrition, it was widely ignored. By securitising the epidemic, the response to HIV/AIDS was elevated to levels never before precipitated by a disease. Four years later, UN Secretary-General Kofi Annan's High-Level Panel on Threats, Challenges and Change submitted a report that would further entrench the notion that health is an issue of collective peace and security. The UN High-Level Panel's report, *A More Secure World: Our Shared Responsibility* listed infectious disease generally, and HIV/AIDS in particular, as an example of a socio-economic threat to security (UN 2004). While framing security as intricately linked to development and human rights, the report seems to evoke the human security continuum of economic, food, health, environmental, personal, community and political issues as threats to stability. The Panel's report argues: 'Any event or process that leads to large-scale death or lessening of life chances and undermines States as the basic unit of the international system is a threat to international security' (UN 2004, 25). The Panel further identified the state as critical to ensuring collective security against threats such as HIV/AIDS.

This is very much in line with activist concepts of human security as conceived by the authors of the UNDP report. In a globalised world, where once distinct material, ideological and geographic boundaries merge and the rights of the poor may affect the lives of the rich, the concept of 'human security' is intended to empower a coalition of people and organisations and to give voice to the numerous non-military threats to the safety of societies in world politics. As such, human security is expected to evoke explicit and emotive discussions, while making empirical observations that are as compelling and practical as possible (Pettman 2005).

Note

1. For example, in the case of a family on an island that is affected by AIDS, most economic models used to project the impact of the epidemic would project that the survivors would enjoy higher per capita income. However, this result neglects the welfare of the family members who died on account of AIDS and the (likely) lower welfare of the surviving members.

References

African Ministers of Defence and Security. 2004. *The African Non-Aggression and Common Defence Pact*. Draft: on the Establishment of the African Standby Force and the Common African Defence and Security Policy, MIN/Def&Sec 4(I), Addis Ababa, 20–21 January 2004, Article 1. The text was adopted during the 2004 African Union (AU) Summit.

Ake, Claude. 1991. 'How Politics Underdevelops Africa'. In *The Challenge of African Economic Recovery and Development*, ed. Adebayo Adedeji, Owodumi Teriba and Patrick Bugembe. Portland: Cass.

———. 1996. *Democracy and Development in Africa*. Washington, DC: Brookings Institution.

Albrow, Martin. 1996. *The Global Age: States and Society beyond Modernity*. Cambridge: Cambridge University Press.

Allen, John and Chris Hamnet (eds.). 1998. *A Shrinking World? Global Unevenness and Inequality*. Oxford: Oxford University Press.

AU (African Union) and UN (United Nations). 2006. 'Africa Launches Bold, Renewed Effort to Step up HIV Prevention'. Addis Ababa, Ethiopia, 12 April. Available at http://www.africa-union.org/News_Events/Newsletter/publication%208.pdf, accessed 25 March 2008.

Bloom, David, David Canning and Dean Jamison. 2004. 'Health, Wealth and Welfare'. *Finance and Development* 41(1), March: 10–15.

Bonnel, Rene. 2000. 'HIV/AIDS: Does it Increase or Decrease Growth? What Makes an Economy HIV-Resistant?' Durban: International AIDS Network Symposium. Available at http://www.ukzn.ac.za/heaRD/publications/publicationsPapers/chapter11.pdf, accessed 25 March 2008.

Booysen, Frederick L.R. and Max Bachmann. 2002. 'HIV/AIDS, Poverty and Growth: Evidence from a Household Impact Study Conducted in the Free State Province, South Africa'. Paper presented at the annual conference of the Centre for the Study of African Economies, St Catherine's College, Oxford, 18-19 March.

Bradshaw, Debbie and Rob Darrington. 2005. 'AIDS-Related Mortality in South Africa'. In *HIV/ AIDS in South Africa*, ed. S.S. Abdool Karim and Q. Abdool Karim, 491-529. Cambridge: Cambridge University Press.

Bratton, Michael and Nicolas van de Walle. 1997. *Democratic Experiments in Africa: Regime Transitions in Comparative Perspective*. Cambridge: Cambridge University Press.

Buzan, Barry. 1991. *People, States and Fear: An Agenda for International Security Studies in the Post-Cold War Era*. Boulder: Lynne Rienner.

————. 2004. 'A Reductionist, Idealistic Notion that Adds Little Analytical Value'. *Security Dialogue* 35(3): 369-70.

Carr, Edward H. 1964. *The Twenty Years' Crisis: 1919-1939*. New York: Harper and Row.

Cheru, Fantu. 1989. *The Silent Revolution in Africa: Debt, Development and Democracy*. London: Zed Books.

Clapham, Christopher. 1996. *Africa and the International System: The Politics of State Survival*. Cambridge: Cambridge University Press.

De Waal, Alex. 2006. *AIDS and Power: Why There Is No Political Crisis – Yet*. Cape Town: David Philip; London and New York: Zed Books.

Dicken, Peter. 1992. *Global Shifts: The Internationalisation of Economic Activity*. London: Paul Chapman.

Donahue, Jill. 1998. *Community-Based Economic Support for Households Affected by HIV/AIDS*. Washington, DC: USAID (United States Agency for International Development), HIV/AIDS Division.

Elbe, Stephen. 2003. *Strategic Implications of HIV/AIDS*. Adelphi Papers, International Institute for Strategic Studies 357.

Engh, Ida-Eline, Libor Stloukal and Jacques du Guerny. 2000. *HIV/AIDS in Namibia: The Impact on the Livestock Sector*. Rome: World Food Programme, Food and Agriculture Organisation.

Fatton, Robert. 1992. *Predatory Rule: State and Civil Society in Africa*. Boulder: Lynne Rienner.

Fukuyama, Francis. 1992. *The End of History and the Last Man*. New York: The Free Press.

Gadamer, Hans Georg. 1983. *Reason in the Age of Science*. Cambridge: Massachusetts Institute of Technology Press.

Giddens, Anthony. 1990. *The Consequences of Modernity*. Cambridge: Polity Press.

Gills, Barry. 1997. 'Globalisation and the Politics of Resistance'. *New Political Economy* 2(1), March: 11-15.

Hosegood, Victoria, Kobus Herbst and Ian Timaeus. 2003. 'The Impact of Adult AIDS Deaths on Households and Children's Living Arrangements in Rural South Africa'. Paper presented at the scientific meeting on 'Empirical Evidence for the Demographic and Socio-Economic Impact of AIDS', hosted by the Health Economics and HIV/AIDS Research Division (HEARD), Durban, 26-28 March.

Huntington, Samuel P. 1996. *The Clash of Civilizations and the Remaking of World Order*. New York: Simon and Schuster.

Iliffe, John. 1995. *Africans: The History of a Continent*. Cambridge: Cambridge University Press.

Kaldor, Mary. 1998. *New and Old Wars: Organised Violence in a Global Era*. Cambridge: Polity Press.

Kennan, George. 1985. 'Morality and Foreign Policy'. *Foreign Affairs* 64(2), 1985–86: 205–18.

Paris, Roland. 2001. 'Human Security; Paradigm Shift or Hot Air?' *International Security* 26(2), Fall: 87–102.

Pettman, Ralph. 2005. 'Human Security as Global Security: Reconceptualising Strategic Studies'. *Cambridge Review of International Affairs* 18(1): 137–50.

Poku, Nana. 1996. 'The Construction of Ethnic Identities in Contemporary Africa'. In *Identities and International Relations*, ed. Neil Renwick and Jill Krause. Basingstoke: Macmillan Press.

——. 2005. *AIDS in Africa: How the Poor are Dying*. Cambridge: Polity Press.

Poku, Nana and David Graham (eds.). 2000. *Migration, Globalisation and Human Security*. London: Routledge.

Poku, Nana and Tony McGrew (eds.). 2007. *Globalisation, Development and Human Security*. Cambridge: Polity Press.

Reno, William. 1998. *Warlord Politics and African States*. Boulder: Lynne Rienner.

Roberts, Adam. 2006. *The Wonga Coup: Guns, Thugs and a Ruthless Determination to Create Mayhem in an Oil-Rich Corner of Africa*. London: Profile Books.

Robertson, Roland. 1992. *Globalisation: Social Theory and Global Culture*. London: Sage.

Steinhauer, Jennifer. 2001. 'UN Redefines Aids as Political Issue and Peril to Poor'. *The New York Times* 28 June.

UN (United Nations). 2004. *A More Secure World: Our Shared Responsibility*. Report of the Secretary-General's High-Level Panel on Threats, Challenges and Change, A/59/565, December.

UNAIDS (Joint United Nations Programme on HIV/AIDS). 2006. 'The Impact of AIDS on People and Societies'. Report on the Global AIDS Epidemic, available at http://www.unaids.org:80/en/KnowledgeCentre/HIVData/GlobalReport/, accessed 7 January 2008.

UNCHGA (United Nations Commission on HIV/AIDS and Governance in Africa). 2004. *HIV/AIDS and Rural Communities*. Addis Ababa: United Nations.

UNDESA (United Nations Department of Economic and Social Affairs). 2005. *The Impact of AIDS*. New York: United Nations.

UNDP (United Nations Development Programme). 1994. *New Dimensions of Human Security*. Human Development Report, available at http://www.hdr.undp.org/reports/global/ 1994/en/, accessed 2 May 2007.

United Nations Department of Peacekeeping Operations. n.d. See http://www.un.org/Depts/dpko/dpko, accessed 18 December 2007.

Waller, Katie. 1998. 'The Impact of HIV/AIDS on Farming Households in the Monze District of Zambia'. Research paper, University of Bath.

Weiss, Herbert and Tatiana Carayannis. 2005. 'The Enduring Idea of the Congo'. In *Borders, Nationalism, and the African State*, ed. Ricardo Rene Laremont. Boulder: Lynne Rienner.

Whiteside, Alan. 2002. 'Poverty and HIV/AIDS in Africa'. *Third World Quarterly* 23(2): 313–32.

Zartman, I. William. 2005. *Cowardly Lions: Missed Opportunities to Prevent Deadly Conflict and State Collapse*. Boulder: Lynne Rienner.

Zartman, I. William (ed.). 1997. *Governance as Conflict Management: Politics and Violence in West Africa*. Washington, DC: Brookings Institute.

2

The Burdens of the Past

———•———

Shula Marks

Introduction

In his comprehensive and judicious history of the African AIDS epidemic, John Iliffe sets out to answer the question posed by South Africa's President Thabo Mbeki: what differentiates the African pandemic from HIV/AIDS elsewhere? Why is it that some two-thirds of the approximately 40 million people living with HIV/AIDS are in Africa, seven times the number in the rest of the world? Iliffe's answer to the apparently rapid spread of the pandemic in Africa is simple: 'Africa', he says, 'had the worst epidemic because it had the first epidemic' (2006, 159).

At an aggregated level, of course, this is true: people living with HIV/AIDS accumulate over the years until those dying of AIDS match or outnumber those newly infected with HIV. This may be happening in some parts of the African continent where the disease is said to be 'stabilising' or 'mature' – a curious choice of terminology for mortality rates that have wiped out all the welfare gains (as reflected in increased life expectancy) of the previous twenty or thirty years.

For South Africa and much of the rest of southern Africa, however, stressing the longevity of the pandemic in Africa does not get us very far. As is often noted, South Africa has the largest number of people living with HIV/AIDS in the world,[1] with more than five million of its adult population infected with the virus. Six countries in the southern African region all have HIV prevalence of more than 20 per cent, while in Swaziland and Botswana, prevalence among adults aged 18–49 is estimated at 33.4 and 24.1 per cent respectively (UNAIDS 2006, 8). However, it should be pointed out that the small populations in Botswana and Swaziland inflate prevalence levels, which are, on the whole, considerably lower than in previous reports, partly as a result of better reporting, partly through the mortality of people living with HIV/AIDS. As the Joint United Nations Programme on HIV/AIDS (UNAIDS) and the World Health Organisation (WHO) remark, southern Africa is 'the epicentre of the global epidemic' (2006a, 10). Yet most of the countries in the region are 'Johnnies come lately' in the grim story of the African epidemic. As late as 1990, the estimated prevalence of HIV/AIDS in South Africa was less than 1 per cent, although the first estimates may have been too low because of under-reporting and under-diagnosis, especially in the rural areas. Today, prevalence is around 18 per cent (with almost one in three pregnant women affected). What is particularly remarkable is the speed with which this has happened: the most dramatic escalation of the pandemic has taken place in the mid-to-late 1990s (Makgoba and Whiteside 2004, 17).

Why South(ern) Africa?

In a highly significant paper, Nicoli Nattrass uses regression analyses to show that today 'simply being a southern African country increases HIV prevalence massively and significantly'. HIV prevalence, she says, 'is *eighteen times* higher for southern African countries' than anywhere else with similar levels of poverty and inequality (n.d.; emphasis in original).[2] This is all the more striking because throughout the 1980s, as South Africans were engaged in the final struggle against apartheid, the country seemed sheltered from the onslaught of a disease that was taking its toll in both developed and developing countries, perhaps because of its relative isolation from the rest of sub-Saharan Africa, especially East Africa, where by the mid-1980s, it was clear that both the rate of increase and the progress of the disease from HIV infection to fully symptomatic AIDS was far more rapid and affected a far broader swathe of society than in the developed world.

The reasons for this are neither entirely clear, nor agreed upon among scientists, and have continued to puzzle President Mbeki. Nevertheless, the existing social science and medical literature does suggest some potential answers. One possibility is that the specific clade, or subtype, of HIV-1 that occurs in southern and eastern Africa, is of greater virulence and infectivity than clades elsewhere.[3] The C clade predominates in southern Africa and Malawi, where HIV/AIDS has proven most devastating. In the Western Cape, with its diverse and historically segregated ethnic groups, both the C clade and the B clade, which is generally found in gay communities in Europe and the Americas, occur, suggesting two separate epidemics.[4] This may contribute to the consistently lower prevalence of HIV/AIDS in the Western Cape.

Whether or not this suggestion is proven correct, the differences in the capacity to control the disease in southern and eastern Africa, both within the C-clade zone, are striking. There is some indication that the epidemic in South Africa has peaked and there has been some behavioural change (for geographical differences, see Actuarial Society of South Africa 2006). Nevertheless, prevalence and incidence levels remain substantially higher in southern than in eastern Africa, despite the considerable private and government resources that have been devoted to preventative programmes on the subcontinent and the ingenuity of non-governmental organisations (NGOs) and civic organisations, especially in South Africa, in tackling such problems as the cost of drugs, denialism and treatment literacy. There is no definitive answer to these challenges, although they suggest the continued need for and force of historical and socio-cultural explanations.

About a decade and a half ago, Anthony Zwi and Antonio Jorge Cabral argued that we needed a new term – they suggested 'high-risk situation' – to describe the range of social, economic and political forces that place groups at particularly high risk of HIV infection (1991). They culled a number of features from a variety of settings in order to characterise these high-risk situations: impoverishment and disenfranchisement, rapid urbanisation, the anonymity of urban life, labour migration, widespread population movements and displacements, and social disruption and wars, especially counter-insurgency wars.[5] They argued that in many of these situations, where daily survival may be precarious and social bonds loosened, there tends to be less worry about healthcare issues and casual sex and more risk-taking behaviour. In these settings, transactional sex (in which sex is exchanged for money or other material support) may represent both a strategy for economic survival and an emotional crutch, and is frequently characterised by highly unequal gender relations; it is also often accompanied by alcohol and drug misuse and high levels of sexually transmitted infections (STIs). Zwi and Cabral's intervention is important because it focused on social conditions, rather than on individual behaviour per se, although recent literature has moved beyond high-risk situations to look at the ways in which behaviour is itself socially determined in these high-risk situations.

In the 1980s, as HIV/AIDS ravaged large parts of East and Central Africa, the first few cases in South Africa were recorded among white homosexual men, on the one hand and Malawian migrant miners, on the other hand, and led initially to great complacency. Black South Africans dismissed HIV/AIDS as 'a white man's disease' and whites blamed it on the promiscuous behaviour of African migrants.

Both groups focused also on other marginalised outsiders – gay men, drug pushers, bisexuals and sex workers. The country was quite unprepared for a generalised crisis as the virus spread from these small, stigmatised groups to the general population. The fact that HIV/AIDS took off in the mid-1990s, as the new post-apartheid government took office, is one of the tragic ironies of South African history.

Yet it took no great prescience to predict that once the virus gained a hold in South Africa the epidemic would be devastating, given the country's inequalities and its underlying burden of disease. By the mid-to-late 1980s, a number of progressive doctors and social scientists were warning that it was simply a matter of time before the epidemic spread from a handful of so-called 'high-risk groups' to the rest of the population, unless drastic action was taken. After all, on any tabulation of high-risk situations, South Africa in the 1980s must have ranked near the top; its black populace was experiencing every one of the high-risk situations cited by Zwi and Cabral (1991).

High-risk situations: Industrialisation and the migrant labour system

Of these high-risk situations, perhaps the most wide-ranging in its effects on both the physical and the psychological well-being of black South Africans was the migrant labour system. Since the mineral discoveries in Kimberley and the Rand in the last third of the nineteenth century, migrant labour has been a defining characteristic of the region and has had an enduring impact on health, family and gender relations, sexuality and violence.

Some fifty years before the appearance of HIV/AIDS in the late twentieth century, Dr Sidney Kark, later to become internationally acclaimed as one of the pioneers of social medicine, and Dr George Gale, Secretary of Health in South Africa between 1946 and 1952, had little doubt that the migrant labour system on which South Africa's industrial revolution was premised was the most important single cause of ill health in the African population.[6] Kark discussed in great detail the deleterious effects of the migrant labour system. The absence of young men from the rural economy as a result of labour migration affected rural well-being through its impact on food production and hence on the nutrition of the community. Migrancy undermined the stability of family life and led to tensions in family relationships and had vast repercussions on public health control, as 'the process of continuous movement of large numbers of people spread a variety of communicable diseases' (Kark 1949, 77–84; see also 1950).[7]

The mines recruited large numbers of men from a wide swathe of southern Africa and exposed them to serious health hazards. Apart from trauma from accidents, which were frequent, these were, most notably, respiratory and STIs. Tuberculosis (TB) and syphilis did not only affect the men themselves; they also infected their families and friends in the rural areas, far beyond the purview of the mine doctors or the state's public health officers. As George Gale pointed out then, and others have pointed out since, however good the healthcare provided for mine workers by their employers, the mining industry did little for miners who developed illnesses once they retired, or for the families who were put at risk by the diseases they brought home with them (see Gale 1943; 1948, 35–39; on Gale more generally, see Marks 2000). Catherine Campbell and Brian Williams put it succinctly: 'The mines effectively externalised many of the long term costs of occupational illnesses which are borne by ex-miners' households and governmental health services in their regions of origin' (1999, 17).

It is of course true that in trying to understand the social context of HIV/AIDS, we need to go beyond 'invoking a crude and undifferentiated role of poverty and/or migrancy' and look at 'the specific interaction of historical, social, political and cultural factors which have shaped the nature of the epidemic'.[8] Nevertheless, given the continued centrality of the mining industry to South Africa's political economy, and with up to 30 per cent of its 250 000-strong workforce currently infected by the virus (Randera 2006), the Kark-Gale analyses of the social and health consequences of migrant labour still have a bearing on the situation in South Africa more than half a century later.[9]

In the late 1990s, Mark Lurie, then a senior researcher at the South African Medical Research Council, described the process graphically:

> If you wanted to spread a sexually transmitted disease, you'd take thousands of young men away from their families, isolate them in single-sex hostels, and give them easy access to alcohol and commercial sex. Then, to spread the disease around the country, you'd send them home every once in a while to their wives and girlfriends. And that's basically the system we have with the mines. (cited in Schoofs 1999)

The fertile soil in which the epidemic took root was prepared by what Kark calls 'the vast social pathological changes' (1949, 83) brought about by the very particular, highly unequal and gendered form taken by South Africa's industrialisation and urbanisation, after the discovery of diamonds and gold in the last third of the nineteenth century.

The social pathology Kark wrote about in the 1940s and 1950s has had the enduring cultural and psycho-social ramifications that he predicted. In the form of racialised capitalism, which developed in the wake of South Africa's mineral revolution, the rewards of industrialisation were (and still are) largely reaped by white people who were considered citizens. The costs, particularly the health costs in this context, were largely borne by black people, who were excluded from citizenship until 1994. For the vast majority, these processes of industrialisation and urbanisation spelt poverty and powerlessness. It is this pattern that laid the basis of the massive inequalities that have characterised South African society historically and continue to do so today. The inequalities between black and white people have been well rehearsed, but those between urban and rural Africans and between men and women have been less frequently addressed.

As progressive public health doctors of the 1940s were well aware, South Africa's industrialisation depended upon the constant movement from all over the sub-continent of large numbers of sexually active, 'single' men from town to countryside and back, the impoverishment of the countryside and the marginalisation of women and children. Not only did this ensure the spread throughout southern Africa of the respiratory infections and STIs acquired on the mines; as we shall see, crucially, the pattern of migrancy also helped to shape the nature of black families, the expression of sexuality and the construction of new gender identities among both men and women. Keith Breckenridge goes so far as to say that it was in the mining industry on the Witwatersrand that 'the ideals and the practice of manhood that have dominated South Africa in this [twentieth] century – what Connell calls hegemonic masculinity – emerged on the mines' (1998, 669).

Although this notion of a single 'hegemonic masculinity' forged on the mines is perhaps a simplification, it is echoed in a groundbreaking study by Catherine Campbell and her colleagues in contemporary Summertown, a gold-mining region in Gauteng province, which looks at the failure of community-based preventive strategies to combat the HIV/AIDS epidemic. Campbell relates this failure to the macho masculine identities underground miners adopt in order to deal with the dangers they face every day in the mines. Underground, she explains, 'real men' must be exceptionally courageous to work under severe conditions and to risk their lives so as to fulfil their obligations as providers. Manhood is inevitably cast as being fearless. Not only does this have its counterpart in the violence of mine culture, as Breckenridge avers; it also shaped male sexual demands – 'associated with this macho masculinity is the notion that a real man has insatiable urges to have sex with an unlimited number of women' (Campbell, Williams and McPhail 1999, 124).

Apartheid and the expansion of the migrant labour system

Despite the warnings of leading public health figures like Kark and Gale against the health hazards of the migrant labour system, in 1948 the newly elected National Party government extended migrancy beyond the mining industry, to all industry within so-called 'white South Africa'. Moreover, from the late 1950s, in pursuit of apartheid policies, the government instigated some of the most massive population movements in peace time, outside of the Soviet Union. Over three million people were uprooted in the heyday of apartheid's social engineering.[10] Settled urban black families were relocated to rural reserves, now referred to as 'Bantu homelands', as were black families living on what were defined as 'white lands'. The 'forty lost years' (O'Meara 1989) between the Nationalists' capture of state power and the transition to democracy were not simply wasted: the changes they wrought ate into the very heart of human relationships, as poverty deepened, communities were destroyed, families disrupted on a vast scale and social norms further eroded.

Contrary to widespread expectation, however, the lifting of measures controlling the influx of Africans into the urban areas in the mid-1980s did not necessarily change things for the better. If anything, the protracted demise of the apartheid regime (which in some sense this signalled) was accompanied by intensified urbanisation, increased violence and further social dislocation (Morris and Hindson 1991). The disintegration of apartheid not only did not end migrant labour, but so deeply entrenched had it become as a mode of survival for rural Africans that the erosion of the state's power of control, together with the impact of economic recession in the 1970s and 1980s and the government's adoption of neoliberal economic policies, accelerated ever larger movements of deeply impoverished people – including large numbers of young single women – into the sprawling shacklands surrounding South Africa's mines and towns. There they became prey to diseases of poverty, such as malnutrition and TB, to parasitic infections and to STIs. The patterns of sexual behaviour that first manifested in the 1930s were re-enacted on a far wider scale.

If the disintegration of apartheid led to a large-scale movement of people, the struggle to end apartheid and the counter-reaction to that struggle took its own toll. The last years of the apartheid regime were characterised by a low-intensity war, unleashed in large measure by the state's so-called 'Third Force', both inside South Africa and across the subcontinent. Although the link between war and the spread of HIV/AIDS has recently been questioned, much depends on the nature of that warfare. Once the virus made its sinister debut, the turmoil in South Africa had few of the isolating effects the conflicts in Angola and northern Uganda are alleged to have had (Dr Peter Ndumbe, personal communication).

This may partly explain why KwaZulu-Natal (KZN) has had such a high prevalence of HIV/AIDS.[11] In addition to the truck routes through the province and the abolition of circumcision among Zulu people in the days of Shaka Zulu, which have both been linked to the province's high HIV/AIDS prevalence, the sexual violence associated with the prolonged, bloody and dirty conflict fought there during the last days of the apartheid regime may have fuelled the epidemic. Perhaps somewhat dramatically, Ashnie Padarath has declared that during this internecine struggle, the 'sexual brutalization of women believed to be supporters of opposing political parties' in KZN was comparable to that in Bosnia in 1992–93 (Padarath 1998, 64; see also Meintjies and Goldblatt 1998).[12] At the same time, in the 1980s and early 1990s, Durban was also the scene of some of the most rapid and disorderly urbanisation on the subcontinent. The long-term oscillation of migrant men was now paralleled by the movement of vulnerable, young, single women into the informal settlements surrounding the towns and mines of South Africa, which were shown to have the highest HIV/AIDS incidence and prevalence, with the possible exception of the mines and the prisons (Shisana and Simbayi 2000, 47).

The heart-stopping euphoria of the 1994 elections, when South Africans cast their votes in a democratic non-racial election for the first time, could not alter the profound economic, social and cultural dislocations of apartheid society, given their scale and historical entrenchment. Nor could it alter the ravaged lungs of the cohorts of miners who returned home with silicosis, which undermined their immune systems and rendered them vulnerable to TB – and possibly also to HIV infection (Marks 2006). Above all, the massive inequalities that characterised South African society under apartheid did not disappear overnight, nor even over the next decade and a half, despite the expansion of a black middle class (Whiteside and Sunter 2000, 61–62). The neoliberal economic policies of the National Party in the 1980s and of the African National Congress (ANC) government post-1994 did little to address these entrenched inequalities and, as in many other parts of the world, may well have exacerbated them. As we shall see, these economic policies also fuelled gender violence.

The continuing war against women

Yet the widespread violence against women has a deeper history, rooted in the social ruptures of twentieth-century South Africa, as work by historians and social scientists over the past decade and a half is beginning to attest.[13]

We have already seen how the migrant labour system was premised on a spatial and gendered definition of work from the outset, as hundreds of thousands of men came to work each year, leaving their wives behind them in the rural reserves, where, at least initially, their agricultural labour subsidised the mines and constituted a form of insurance for returning migrants. A gendered division of labour and a gender and age hierarchy, in which women were subordinate to men, characterised African rural society and articulated well with the patriarchy of settler society and the demand for male labour in the mines. In the all-male compounds on the mines, more experienced and older men exercised sexual (and other) power over their juniors through the metaphor of gender (Moodie, Ndatshe and Sibuye 1988, 228–42; Harries 1990, 318–36).

Moreover, linked to the 'startling absence of women from the social life of the mines' and related to it, was the ubiquity of violence underground (Breckenridge 1998, 669). Again this drew on an established tradition of contained aggression among young men in the rural areas, in common with that among most young men in most cultures. There was, however, more to violence on the mines, which Breckenridge suggests 'was an essential part of the definition of racial identities, and the practical force of racist hierarchy underground. But it was also a celebrated, and defining, ideal of masculinity for both white and black men.' (1998, 669)

While the hierarchy and discipline of the mines held some of these explosive tensions at bay, already early in the twentieth century, African Christian mothers, African chiefs, missionaries and government officials were expressing their concern about the impact of migrant labour on the purity of young girls in the rural areas, who were subjected to intolerable pressures when the men returned home. At the same time, older forms of sex education and modes of contraception already denigrated by colonial conquest, conversion and the missionary onslaught on initiation practices (the arena for sexual socialisation in many pre-colonial societies), were lost as a result of family disruption and labour migrancy, and not replaced.[14] Ironically, in view of the predilection of many commentators to see promiscuity and violence as a primordial fact of African life, it was often the Christian families that first experienced the higher rates of premarital pregnancy that resulted. Peter Delius and Clive Glaser put it succinctly: 'Christian morality and the pursuit of modernity [which frequently accompanied and even encouraged conversion] made a potent cocktail which stigmatised traditional forms of restraint but failed to curb the heightened sexual impulses of pubescent youth' (2002, 36).

By the 1930s, what had first affected Christian converts had generalised to confront all African communities on the subcontinent as labour migrancy spread its tentacles. For young men, whether Christian or not, 'the harsh and often violent world of the compound, the hostel, the *amalaita* gangs and even the prison' became the new context for sexual socialisation. In these new spaces, the sanctions curbing male aggression also loosened and many communities experienced 'an upward spiral of violence', not simply between young men themselves, but also very specifically against women (Delius and Glaser 2002, 38).

Anne Mager, for example, has poignantly described how, in the Eastern Cape by the 1930s and 1940s, sexuality and violence had become fatally linked.[15] Using court records of the time, she argues that in the Ciskei 'violence was escalating, fast becoming "like a war on women"' (1995, 203–05; 1996, 2). She sees this 'war on women' (a phrase that has since become something of a cliché among contemporary journalists) as the result of broader economic, social and political forces intermingling with gender inequalities. The 'crisis in the gendered ordering of African society' was, she says, in part, 'the outcome of desperate attempts by African men to reassert patriarchal domination in a rapidly changing world' (1996, 2), and in part, the result of a decline in the economic importance of women's fertility. As a consequence, women came increasingly to be regarded as sexual objects for male pleasure. In these circumstances, 'girls and their bodies were under enormous pressure from lustful men. Educated middle class men entrusted with responsibility for young girls and boys often failed to set an example of self-restraint. Some used their positions for personal gratification . . . There were . . . instances of male teachers and policemen engaging in sex with pupils.' (1996, 2) As we have seen above, violence against young girls, many of them school children, continues to this day.[16] Mager concludes:

> In a context of absent male migrants, economic hardship, personal
> insecurity and political emasculation, sexual violence became endemic
> . . . In a context where male power was constructed around control
> over women, male aggression was readily expressed, often blurring the
> line between assault and sexuality for both men and women . . . Sexual
> violence was an outlet for power and anger; it was an expression of
> masculinities that depended on the submission of women. (1996, 16)

From this and other accounts, it is clear that the 'hegemonic masculinity' of the
mines (Breckenridge 1998, 669), itself in part derived from earlier ideals of male
behaviour, accompanied the biological pathogens and dust particles from mine
and compound along the migrant routes back home to the rural areas. It also spilt
over into the burgeoning towns of the late 1930s and 1940s, intersecting with an
older gang culture with its own larger-than-life claims of manhood in the 1930s and
1940s. Delius and Glaser describe this well: 'Denied the traditional route to
adulthood, gang members tried to compensate with displays of physical strength,
violence and daring. The gang subculture awarded status to multiple sexual
conquests. Criminal activity often allowed for conspicuous spending to lure women,
tsotsis competed furiously for the most attractive girls.' (2002, 44) More widely,
urban teenage sexual expression was now no longer bound by earlier peer and
parental constraints. From the 1930s, as young unattached women came into the
cities, the 'conjunction of deprived men and unattached women in a tight-packed
urban slum' led to far freer sexual relationships, and 'men certainly expected full
intercourse and often beat girlfriends who denied them' (Mayer 1961, 252 cited in
Delius and Glaser 2002, 45). While the timing varied from place to place, 'the
patterns of sexual behaviour . . . were similar': the breakdown of parental control
and peer groups opened the way to the premarital pregnancies that earlier
socialisation practices had so carefully controlled (Delius and Glaser 2002, 45–46).

If the groundwork for a new sexual order was laid by the mid-twentieth century,
it was further developed and entrenched in the heyday of apartheid. Furthermore,
the struggles of the comrades that led to apartheid's demise in no way challenged
the often violent masculinity that had evolved among the youth in the gangs on the
streets of the locations. As has been frequently noted, '*Comrade* culture was highly
masculinist' and women were increasingly marginalised (Delius and Glaser 2002,

48), as were parents and teachers, whose authority had been undermined by the youth politics of the 1980s. By the time of the 1994 elections, one could argue that there was a multiplicity of masculine identities, with shifting boundaries, but generally sharing many of the characteristics of the 'hegemonic masculinity' forged in the mines (Breckenridge 1998, 669).

Since 1994: Four vignettes

The success of the struggle against apartheid and the entrenchment of one of the most gender-sensitive Constitutions in the world could do little to diminish deeply held beliefs about appropriate masculine behaviour that had been forged over the previous century and more of conquest, exploitation and impoverishment. The legacies of the past and the continued neoliberalism of the present have deeply scarred post-apartheid South Africa. The violence that characterised the last days of apartheid and the structural deformations that preceded it have not disappeared, as the extraordinary crime statistics attest (in this context, especially statistics for rape and violence against women and children). As Mamphela Ramphele has recognised: 'The end of apartheid has not necessarily changed the reality of many poor men. Their only escape from complete powerlessness is the control they exercise over African women and children. It is not surprising that some of them become abusive of their own children and the women in their lives.' (2000, 114) Meredeth Turshen puts it even more strongly: 'Violence and the threat of violence against women do not end with peace accords [or, one might add, gender-sensitive Constitutions]: the violence of a regime begets a general culture of violence. In South Africa, murder, rape and assaults are now both a cultural and statistical norm.' (Turshen and Twagiramariya 1998, 9)

The exact statistics for rape and violence against women in South Africa (as elsewhere) cannot be known, but what is clear from numerous studies is the high degree of coercive sex experienced by its women (and some men) – both black and white (see, for example, Dempster 2002). The country is said to have the highest per capita number of *reported* rape cases in the world, not infrequently perpetrated against children and even babies. The numbers can only be described as horrifying: in December 2000, 13 540 children under the age of seventeen were raped, of whom almost 8 000 were under the age of eleven.[17] This means that in South Africa, a child is abused every 8 minutes, a child is assaulted every 14 minutes and a child is raped every 24 minutes of the day and night (POWA n.d.). And, it is widely agreed, these numbers probably only represent the tip of the iceberg. We should not perhaps be surprised that in the wake of the HIV/AIDS epidemic, public confessionals by the Truth and Reconciliation Commission (TRC) and these statistics, sexuality in South Africa has become highly politicised (Posel 2005a).

Increased press attention may have heightened popular perceptions that rape has increased dramatically since 1994, but whether they represent an increase or not, the figures are shocking. People Opposing Women Abuse (POWA), which began collecting the statistics in the 1980s, claimed in 2002 that one in two South African women could be raped in her lifetime, that a woman is raped every 26 seconds, murdered by 'an intimate partner' every six days, and that 25 per cent of women have suffered domestic abuse (POWA n.d.; see also Palitza 2005). To its credit, the government has recognised the gravity of the issue and has made considerable resources available to tackle it, but as yet, there is no evidence to suggest that this has had much impact. Iliffe's magisterial *The African AIDS Epidemic*, which I cited at the beginning of this chapter, is curiously almost silent on what must surely rank as one of the critical causes of human insecurity in South Africa and an important, if as yet insufficiently analysed, factor in the spread of HIV/AIDS.[18]

It is, of course, true that the causal links between rape and other forms of domestic violence are not totally clear. Nevertheless, as Lisa Vetten and Khailash Bhana suggest, there are at least four major plausible hypotheses linking HIV/AIDS with rape and other forms of sexual abuse – quite apart from the intrinsic suffering and trauma that result from it. These hypotheses are: the violence of rape and other forms of coerced sex frequently leads to female genital injury (which facilitates the transmission of HIV/AIDS); while assault by multiple assailants in gang rape also compounds risk; both rape and non-physical abuse limit women's ability to insist on condom use; childhood sexual abuse may lead to riskier sexual behaviour later on; and women whose HIV status becomes known are often subjected to abuse by their partners, and even, on occasion, murder (Vetten and Bhana 2001).

The current epidemic of rape and violence against women has also been explained as part of the violence already permeating contemporary South African society. More specifically, as a number of authors have observed, this gendered violence reflects a crisis around male identity as unemployment numbers have soared, and as neither marriage nor even casual transactional sex are options often open to the poorest of poor men in post-apartheid South Africa.[19] It may also be exacerbated by the suspicions roused by the HIV/AIDS epidemic, as Vetten and Bhana argue. That the response should be expressed in high levels of violence against women needs further explanation, however.

Windows on the epidemic

Recent case studies provide windows onto the ways in which the neoliberal economic policies adopted by the National Party government in the 1980s and early 1990s and continued by the ANC-led government have reshaped sexual identities and influenced the spread of the HIV/AIDS pandemic in contemporary South Africa. Here a few examples must suffice.

The so-called single-sex hostels in Cape Town, studied by Ramphele in the 1980s, illustrate masculinities that were based on the subordination of women and the diffusion of these masculinities far beyond the mines or men's rural hinterlands. She stresses the way in which male violence against women was an outcome of the exploitation and subordination of men in apartheid society and their wider lack of power or control. In the hostels of the Cape Flats, she argues, black men were able to exert their power over the only individuals in a weaker position than they were: the women who were in town illegally and were dependent on them for a bed, food and income, as well as an often double-edged 'protection' (Ramphele 1993).

Mark Hunter's study of Isithebe, an informal settlement in KZN with twice the national average of HIV/AIDS prevalence, complicates, but does not jettison, the migrant labour narrative (2006). Like Ramphele, he suggests that the high prevalence of HIV/AIDS in urban shacklands like Isithebe has to be located in South Africa's changing political economy from the 1970s. With rising unemployment and falling wages, men could no longer afford *ilobolo* (bridewealth) for marriage and increasing numbers of young women came to town on their own in search of a livelihood. For many, sex work was the only possible means of survival. Without kin and few resources, Hunter argues, they were particularly vulnerable in an age of HIV/AIDS in which multiple partners, high rates of STIs and male antipathy to condoms fuelled the pandemic.

In the Limpopo province, Isak Niehaus suggests a somewhat different impetus for the 'war on women'. Here, he argues, the usual explanation that rape is simply a demonstration of masculine power applies only to sexual intimidation by fairly socially advantaged men (2002). Young rural men without access even to migrant labour (and there is one thing worse than migrant labour – no labour at all), are not only unable to find the *ilobolo* for marriage and thus full initiation into adulthood, they are also unable to afford the casual sex available to those with money or gifts to offer. The escalation of extreme poverty in the last couple of decades has thus changed the dynamic of sexual coercion. From the evidence he has garnered from detailed 'sexual biographies of young men' in the former rural reserve of Bushbuckridge in the 1990s, Niehaus suggests that in the time of 'de-industrialisation', 'marginal men who fell well short of meeting masculine ideals were more likely to perpetrate rape . . . rape can [thus] also be seen as a violent attempt to symbolically assert – and sometimes even mimic – a dominant masculine persona. Through rape men demonstrate their heterosexual virility, humiliate economically successful women or enact an idea of patriarchal rule within households.' (Niehaus 2002; 2005) Like Hunter, Niehaus believes that to understand the dramatic increase in the number of rapes in South Africa in the last twenty years, it is essential to acknowledge the local complexities of the phenomenon, as well as its broader political and economic context in a rapidly changing country.

This is undoubtedly true. Nevertheless, there is a certain over-determination in the actual manifestation of male insecurities in violence against women in contemporary South Africa. The social pathology that Kark observed in the 1940s and 1950s and the 'hegemonic masculinity' that Breckenridge discerned as emanating from the mines do seem to have had enduring cultural and psycho-social ramifications. While present-day violence and its relationship to HIV/AIDS has to be understood in the context of the contemporary political economy and cannot simply read off the past, equally there seems to be a template of responses that are used over and over again in different contexts and circumstances and for different reasons. Neither the context of a changing political economy, however, nor the template of responses derived from the past removes the need to understand violence under the particular circumstances of its expression in particular spaces and with particular meanings. Only in this way can we begin to understand the protean ways in which HIV both shapes and is shaped by its entry into very specific ethnographic niches, themselves the product of specific historical experience, a changing political economy and contemporary exigencies.

Moreover, as important as the *longue durée* has been in inculcating certain forms of hegemonic masculinity, hegemony is never total: it is always both incomplete and contested. There were and are alternate models of both male and female behaviour and very different overlapping and competing sexual identities, some of the more creative emerging in the very crucible of the HIV/AIDS pandemic itself.

Enticing as it is, the notion of hegemonic masculinity also needs to be unravelled, so as to avoid relying on singular models, which are reductionist constructs that do not account for material, psychological and cultural realities.

So far, most of the emphasis in this chapter has been on men. Faced with the bleak statistics of violence against women, it is easy to see them simply as passive victims, accepting of male domination and without agency of their own. Yet women, too, respond to the realities of their material life, making choices, however circumscribed and even potentially fatal, under circumstances not of their choosing (see Chapter 4 in this volume). Suzanne Leclerc-Madlala provides a useful corrective. She says that in the globally connected, consumerist world that exists in the midst of poverty in contemporary South Africa's metropolitan areas, prostitution and survival sex do not adequately describe forms of sexual exchange in which young women are not passive victims, but rather active as agents in the manipulation of their sexual partners, in order to access a more sophisticated lifestyle and the goods that accompany this status (2003).

Such 'sex for money exchanges', often with multiple partners, are clearly very different to the economic necessity that drives sexual encounters in the desolate landscape of the mines and informal settlements of South Africa. Nevertheless, these practices too, are linked to 'high rates of HIV infection and high levels of social acceptance of violence against women' (Wojcicki 2002 cited in Leclerc-Madlala 2003, 217; see also Hunter 2002). In Leclerc-Madlala's study in Durban, young women were well aware of the dangers of unprotected sex with multiple partners. Confronted with the deaths of friends and relatives, however, the fear that they were also at risk drove their efforts to gain access to material well-being while they still could (2003).

These local case studies are not simply anecdotal; they suggest the vital importance of *disaggregating* the HIV/AIDS prevalence statistics in southern Africa and engaging with people's subjective meanings and the way they construct their sexuality, if the attempts to stem the disease through prevention and treatment are to have any hope of success. Paradoxically, while HIV/AIDS is both the ultimate global disease, which has to be 'framed within the context of the wider global processes that impact on health and health care in Africa in which the international community is deeply implicated', it demands, at the same time, the closest attention to the specificity of the social and cultural circumstances that shape individual behaviour (Campbell 2003, 193).

Unheeded warnings

Given its history, it is clear from the analysis so far that South Africa was unlikely to have escaped the HIV/AIDS pandemic, however far-sighted its medics, however determined its political leaders. This said, however, the *extent* of the spread of the virus was far from inevitable: with vision and determination, it may have been possible to contain the epidemic in its early stages. This was recognised in 1989 at a historic meeting in Zimbabwe between the ANC in exile and members of the progressive medical association, the National Medical and Dental Association (NAMDA). Among the commissions set up to report to the meeting was a special panel on HIV/AIDS, which included contributions from medical personnel in South Africa, the United Kingdom and the United States. Ominously foreshadowing later developments, in introducing the discussion on the report, the chairperson pointed out that 6 per cent of teenage girls in (then) Natal attending a clinic for sexually transmitted diseases had recently tested HIV positive (NAMDA 1990, 20). In its report, the panel acknowledged that the epidemic was 'already a problem of massive proportions. At this stage it is not possible to defeat the HIV virus, but it would be possible to contain it. We have to assume a wide spread already, because it takes 5–10 years before the cases will present in clinical form.' (1990, 19) Arguing that among the many factors that made it more difficult to combat the disease was the apartheid government's lack of legitimacy and its failure to tackle the disease, the meeting urged 'the Movement'[20] to do so. The panel ended its report by quoting from a paper by Dr Sam Couston:

> In South Africa it is self evident that the [apartheid] government is completely lacking in the credibility necessary to influence sexual behaviour in the black community. The only political organisations which have that credibility among the majority of South African people are the liberation movements, internal and external. It is my greatest fear and recurring nightmare, that I will go to South Africa after Independence and find the wards of the hospitals full of AIDS patients, the new country burdened with the morbidity, mortality and expense of an AIDS epidemic indefinitely. In one sense you are uniquely fortunate in knowing enough, early enough, to prevent this. But the time to act is now. And you are the people who must act. (NAMDA 1990, 21)

Unfortunately, the grim story of HIV/AIDS in South Africa is also a tragic story of missed opportunities and needless loss of life. Almost overwhelmed by the enormity of the tasks before it, the post-1994 government first ignored this message and then obfuscated. Far from learning from the past and from experiences in the rest of sub-Saharan Africa, the new government paid little more attention to its progressive medics than the apartheid government had done in 1948.[21] Perhaps reluctant to engage with the intimate complexities of sexuality, perhaps unable to accept the full horror confronting them, South Africa's leadership has only recently, as a result of the intervention of the former Deputy-Minister of Health, Nozizwe Madlala-Routledge and the Deputy-President, Phumzile Mlambo-Ngcuka, begun to take serious account of the devastating consequences of the pandemic, to resuscitate the South African National AIDS Council and to engage with civic organisations to ensure the roll-out of life-saving antiretroviral (ARV) drugs and treatment literacy (see, for example, Bevan 2006a, 2006b; see also National Civil Society HIV/AIDS Conference 2006).

These movements towards a more whole-hearted engagement with the epidemic, though, were stalled by President Mbeki's dismissal of Madlala-Routledge in August 2007, to the outrage of activists (see SAPA 2007). Hopes of more progressive HIV policy implementation were raised again with the election of Jacob Zuma to the ANC presidency in December 2007,[22] but the effects of this election on HIV policy, if any, have yet to unfold.

Conclusion: Where do we go from here?
Confronted by these historical legacies and contemporary realities of government foot-dragging and worse, it is perhaps understandable that at times even the most optimistic feel despair. Nevertheless, however belatedly, the end of 2006 did seem to have witnessed a change of direction on the part of government and gave some room for cautious optimism that at last the government is turning its back on the years of obfuscation – too late for the hundreds of thousands who have already died, but offering some hope for the presently afflicted. There is general agreement on the seriousness of the problem, the scale of the pandemic and the urgent need to scale up ARV treatment.

Even more important in encouraging a cautious optimism is the myriad of NGOs – most notably Médecins san Frontières (MSF) and the Treatment Action Campaign (TAC) – and grassroots organisations that have pioneered innovative and imaginative ways of addressing the epidemic in the face of government neglect, if not hostility. The TAC, led by the indefatigable and indomitable Zackie Achmat, has provided inspiration not only to the thousands of people living with HIV/AIDS in South Africa, but to their counterparts all over the world. If this compassion, vision, energy and determination can now engage with the new problems to be solved – the establishment of appropriate health structures, treatment literacy campaigns and realistic programmes of prevention – a new and more constructive era may yet be about to unfold in South Africa.

Notes

1. The absolute numbers in India were once predicted to be greater than those in South Africa, but relative to the size of population, HIV prevalence is far lower in India.

2. I am grateful to Dr Nattrass for allowing me to quote from her paper and for explaining her methodology to a novice. Logistic regression tables help one to determine which explanatory variables are independent predictors. Nattrass initially used two variables: (the log of) per capita income and the Gini co-efficient (a measure of social inequality), which have been regarded as predictive of the variance in HIV prevalence (see, for example, Barnett and Whiteside 1999, 200–34). The difference between the predicted value and the actual value for HIV prevalence (which, in the southern African case is considerable) is thus a measure of what the model is *not* able to explain. Nattrass shows that by including a 'dummy variable' in a new regression, which takes the value of one if the country is a southern African country, one can explain a lot more of the variation in HIV prevalence worldwide. 'Put differently' she says, 'simply being a Southern African country [vastly] increases the explained proportion of South Africa's HIV prevalence . . .' (e-mail communication, 13 April 2005).

3. I am grateful to Dr Peter Ndumbe of Cameroon for alerting me to this possibility (personal communication, 8 February 2008).

4. There are two main types of the HI virus: HIV-1 and HIV-2. HIV-2 is mainly found in West Africa and is known to have a longer incubation period and is less easily transmitted through mother-to-child transmission than HIV-1. HIV-1 has been divided into two main groups: O for Outliers (mainly Gabon, Cameroon and France) and M for Main group, which is further subdivided into at least eight clades or subtypes, designated by letters. South Africa has both B and C clades.

5. Recent research suggests, perhaps counter-intuitively, that war and displacement do not necessarily lead to a higher risk of contracting HIV/AIDS, especially where the populace is rendered immobile and relatively isolated. See Spiegel and Haroff-Tavel (2006) and Fabiani et al. (2006) in the UNAIDS/WHO 'Aids Epidemic Update' (2006).

6. I have discussed their views more fully elsewhere; see Marks 2002.

7. One should note that while I have simply referred to Sidney Kark here, Emily Kark may well have alerted him to the social implications of migrant labour.

8. This was the caveat issued by the organisers of the conference, 'HIV AIDS in Social Context', held at the University of the Witwatersrand, Johannesburg, in 2001.

9. The number of miners dropped from over 500 000 in the late 1980s to half of this number by the late 1990s. However, in the 1990s, there were between two and three million legal migrants working in South Africa's mines, farms and factories, quite apart from those working illegally in the country.

10. For estimates of the numbers and the laws involved in the population removals under apartheid, see The Surplus People's Project (1983a, 1983b). For the estimated number of people removed between 1960 and 1982, see Table 1 in The Surplus People's Project (1983a, 6).

11. Recent research has shown that circumcision gives considerable (although not total) protection against infection (see Reuters 2006). It should be noted that the *Household Survey* (Shisana and Simbayi 2002) found rather lower prevalence statistics for KZN to those based on data from antenatal clinics – which by definition deal with the sexually active; as the authors point out, most of the clinics are close to the major transport routes, where incidence tends to be higher. HIV prevalence is now lower in KZN than it was because, as Shisana and Simbayi show, there has been some behaviour change (2002, 46). As the first province to be hit by the epidemic, it has had the highest mortality. Nevertheless, according to the Department of Health (2000, 8), the prevalence of HIV/AIDS in pregnant women in KZN in 2000 was 32.5 per cent, while the Actuarial Society's 'Report on the State of the South African HIV/AIDS Epidemic' (2006) still shows the highest prevalence in KZN.

12. The analogy with Bosnia, where rape seems to have been deliberately adopted as war policy, while thought-provoking, is not wholly valid. There is no way of knowing the absolute numbers of women raped either in Bosnia between 1992 and 1995 (which have ranged from 20 000 to 100 000) or in KZN during the decade-long conflict (1984–94), although given the population statistics (themselves guesstimates) the incidence seems to have been far higher in Bosnia.

13. I discussed some of this in an earlier paper (see Marks 2002). In addition to the bibliographical note there, there is exciting new work, especially on masculinity (see, for example, Morrell 1998, 2001). Also see the essays that came out of 'Sex and Secrecy', the 4th International Conference of the Association for the Study of Sexuality, Culture and Society held at the University of the Witwatersrand in 2003. Many of the papers presented there are included in Reid and Walker's excellent collection, *Men Behaving Differently? South African Men since 1994* (2005). The spate of academic literature mirrors the extraordinary transformation in public discourse remarked on by Posel (2005b, 125–53).

14. For a pioneering historical exploration of sexual socialisation in pre-colonial and early colonial African societies, see Delius and Glaser (2002) and Gaitskell (1982).

15. Most of my citations are taken from Mager (1996) because this is the most succinct statement of her views, although I have also used Mager (1995). The substance is identical to that of her book on gender in the Ciskei (1999).

16. On the rape of children, see Mager (1996). For the rape of school girls specifically, see Department of Education (2000), cited in Human Rights Watch (2001, 36). It is estimated that school teachers

are responsible for about one-third of rapes committed against young girls in contemporary South Africa.

17. The evidence on child rape and especially the rape of babies with its fearful physical consequences has shocked South Africans. As Rachel Jewkes (2002) has pointed out, the role of the widely cited belief that having sex with a virgin cures AIDS in childhood rape has probably been exaggerated; this does not, however, reduce the horror of the phenomenon.

18. It is in his silences on gender inequality that Iliffe's book is most flawed. Revealingly, when you look up 'gender' in the index, you are directed to look under 'women'. This is somewhat better than his treatment of racism, masculinity, rape and violence. Most of these issues and their relationship to HIV/AIDS receive little attention in his text and none of them merit an index entry.

19. The link between abject poverty, unemployment, gang culture and rape is evident also in Haiti, which would seem to have similar levels of rape and other forms of violence against women (see Renton 2007). According to Renton, people in Haiti explained rape as 'the result of the lack of policing, proper governance, unemployment and the failed economy . . . part of the general breakdown of society' (55).

20. 'The Movement' is generally a euphemism for the ANC, but in the 1980s, it could also denote the tacit coalition between the ANC, the Mass Democratic Movement and the Congress of South African Trade Unions (COSATU).

21. The South African government is not unique in this. As De Waal has pointed out in his exceptionally lucid and informative recent book, *AIDS and Power* (2006), most African governments have been able to 'manage' rather than 'prevent' the 'catastrophe' of HIV/AIDS in large measure because their publics do not demand or even expect government action in the face of the disease.

22. TAC chairman Zackie Achmat reacted to Zuma's election, saying, 'For the first time there is a glasnost in our country, and that makes us excited' (see Reuters 2007).

References

Actuarial Society of South Africa. 2006. 'Summary of Biennial Report on the State of the South African HIV/AIDS Epidemic'. Available at http://www.doh.gov.za/docs/reports/2006/summary.html, accessed 13 February 2007.

Barnett, Tony and Gwyn Prins. 2006. *AIDS and Security: Fact, Fiction and Evidence: A Report to UNAIDS*. London: London School of Economics.

Barnett, Tony and Alan Whiteside. 1999. 'HIV/AIDS and Development: Case Studies and a Conceptual Framework'. *The European Journal of Development Research* 11(2), December: 200–34.

Bevan, Stephan. 2006a. 'African Minister Ends Decade of Denial on AIDS'. *The Telegraph* 11 December. Available at http://www.telegraph.co.uk, accessed 8 January 2008.

———. 2006b. 'Aids Confusion Catches up Manto and Mbeki'. *Sunday Tribune* 10 December. Available at http://www.iol.co.za, accessed 8 January 2008.

Breckenridge, Keith. 1998. 'The Allure of Violence: Men, Race and Masculinity on the South African Goldmines, 1900–1950'. *Journal of Southern African Studies* 24: 669–93.

Campbell, Catherine. 2003. *Letting Them Die: Why HIV/AIDS Intervention Programmes Fail*. Oxford: James Currey; Indiana: Indian University Press; New York: Double Storey.

Campbell, Catherine and Brian Williams. 1999. 'Responses to HIV/AIDS in the Mining Industry: Past Experiences and Future Challenges'. In *Managing HIV/AIDS in South Africa: Lessons from Industrial Settings*, ed. Brian Williams, Catherine Campbell and Catherine McPhail. Johannesburg: CSIR (Council for Scientific and Industrial Research).

Campbell, Catherine, Brian Williams and Catherine McPhail. 1999. *Managing HIV/AIDS in South Africa: Lessons from Industrial Settings*. Johannesburg: CSIR.

De Waal, Alex. 2006. *AIDS and Power: Why There Is No Political Crisis – Yet*. London and New York: Zed Books; Cape Town: David Philip.

Delius, Peter and Clive Glaser. 2002. 'Sexual Socialisation in South Africa: A Historical Perspective'. *African Studies* 61(1): 27–54.

Dempster, Carolyn 2002. 'Rape – Silent War on SA Women'. *BBC News Online* 9 April. Available at news.bbc.co.uk/1/hi/world/africa/1909220.stm, accessed 8 January 2008.

Department of Education. 2000. 'Message from the Minister of Education'. In *The HIV/AIDS Emergency Guidelines for Educators*. Pretoria: Department of Education.

DoH (Department of Health). 2000. *HIV and AIDS/STD Strategic Plan for South Africa 2000–2005*. Cape Town: Government Printer. Available at http://www.doh.gov.za/aids/docs/aids-plan/, accessed 8 January 2008.

Fabiani, Massimo, Barbara Nattabi, Chiara Pierotti, Filippo Ciantia, Alex A. Opio, Joshua Musinguzi, Emintone O. Ayella and Silvia Declich. 2006. 'HIV-1 Prevalence and Factors Associated with Infection in the Conflict-Affected Region of North Uganda'. Abstract C15, presented at the 16th International Aids Conference in Toronto, Canada, 13–18 August.

Gaitskell, Deborah. 1982. 'Wailing for Purity: Prayer Unions, African Mothers and Adolescent Daughters, 1912–1940'. In *Industrialisation and Social Change: African Class Formation, Culture and Consciousness, 1870–1930*, ed. Shula Marks and Richard Rathbone. London and New York: Longman.

Gale, George. 1943. 'Falling off in Native Health: Evidence before the [Lansdowne] Commission'. *The Star* 11 October.

———. 1948. 'Evidence before the Fagan Commission, U.G. 28-'48, the Union of South Africa'. *Report of the Native Laws Commission*. Pretoria: Government Stationer.

Harries, Patrick. 1990. 'Symbols and Sexuality: Culture and Identity in the Early Witwatersrand Gold Mines'. *Gender and History* 2: 318–36.

Human Rights Watch. 2001. 'Scared at School: Sexual Violence against Girls in South African Schools'. New York: Human Rights Watch. Available at http://www.hrw.org/reports/pdfs/c/crd/za-final.pdf, accessed 25 January 2007.

Hunter, Mark. 2002. '"The Materiality of Everyday Sex": Thinking beyond Prostitution'. *African Studies* 61(1): 99–120.

———. 2006. 'Informal Settlements as Spaces of Health Inequality: The Changing Economic and Spatial Roots of the AIDS Pandemic, from Apartheid to Neo-liberalism'. Research Report 44. University of KwaZulu-Natal: Centre for Civil Society.

Iliffe, John. 2006. *The African Aids Epidemic: A History*. Athens, Ohio: Ohio University Press; Oxford: James Currey; Cape Town: Double Storey (Juta).

Jewkes, Rachel. 2002. 'The Virgin Myth and Child Rape in South Africa'. MRC News release reported in *Science in Africa*, April. Available at http://www.scienceinafrica.co.za/2002/april/rape.htm, accessed 4 January 2007.

Kark, Sidney. 1949. 'The Social Pathology of Syphilis in Africans'. *South African Medical Journal* 23(5), 29 January: 77–84.

———. 1950. 'The Influence of Urban-Rural Migration on Bantu Health and Disease'. *The Leech*, November.

Leclerc-Madlala, Suzanne. 2003. 'Transactional Sex and the Pursuit of Modernity'. *Social Dynamics* 29: 1–21.

Mager, Anne. 1995. 'Gender and the Making of the Ciskei, 1945–1959'. Ph.D. diss., University of Cape Town.

———. 1996. 'Sexuality, Fertility and Male Power in the Eastern Cape'. Unpublished seminar paper, presented to the seminar on the Societies of Southern Africa, 7 November. London: Institute of Commonwealth Studies.

———. 1999. *Gender and the Making of a South African Bantustan: A Social History of the Ciskei, 1945–1959*. Cape Town: Heinemann.

Makgoba, Malegapuru William and Alan Whiteside. 2004. 'HIV/AIDS: Confronting the Future in Southern Africa'. 2003 Canon Collins Memorial Lecture. London: CCETSA (Canon Collins Educational Trust for Southern Africa).

Marks, Shula. 2000. 'George Gale, Social Medicine and the State in South Africa'. In *Science and Society in South Africa*, ed. Saul Dubow. Manchester: Manchester University Press.

———. 2002. 'An Epidemic Waiting to Happen? The Spread of HIV/AIDS in South Africa in Social and Historical Perspective'. *African Studies* 61(1): 13–26.

———. 2006. 'The Silent Scourge? Silicosis, Respiratory Disease and Gold-Mining in South Africa'. *Journal of Ethnic and Migration Studies* 32(4) (May): 569–89.

Mayer, Philip. 1961. *Townsmen of Tribesmen: Conservatism and the Process of Urbanization in a South African City*. Cape Town: Oxford University Press.

Meintjies, Sheila and Beth Goldblatt. 1998. 'South African Women Demand the Truth'. In *What Women Do in War Time: Gender and Conflict in Africa*, ed. Meredeth Turshen and Clotilde Twagiramariya. New York: Zed Books.

Moodie, T. Dunbar, Vivien Ndatshe and British Sibuye. 1988. 'Migrancy and Male Sexuality on the South African Gold Mines'. *Journal of Southern African Studies* 14(2): 228–42.

Morrell, Robert (ed.). 1998. *Journal of Southern African Studies* 24(4), December. Special issue on 'Masculinities in Southern Africa'.

———. 2001. *Changing Men in Southern Africa*. Pietermaritzburg: University of Natal Press; London: Zed Books.

Morris, Mike and Doug Hindson. 1991. 'Political Violence and Urban Reconstruction in South Africa'. Unpublished paper for the Economic Trends meeting, 17 July.

NAMDA (National Medical and Dental Association). 1990. *NAMDA Special Bulletin 3*. February. NAMDA-ANC meeting 21–22 October 1989, held in Harare, Zimbabwe. Congella, Durban: NAMDA Publications.

National Civil Society HIV/AIDS Conference. 2006. 'A Victory for Civil Society Activism'. Conference held 27-28 October in Randburg. Available at http://www.sangonet.org.za, accessed 4 January 2007.

Nattrass, Nicoli. n.d. 'AIDS, Inequality and Access to Antiretroviral Treatment: A Comparative Analysis'. In *New Departures in Political Science*, ed. Ian Shapiro. New Haven: Yale University, forthcoming.

Niehaus, Isak. 2002. 'Renegotiating Masculinity in the South African Lowveld'. *African Studies* 61(1), 1 July: 77-97.

———. 2005. 'Masculine Domination in Sexual Violence: Interpreting Accounts of Three Cases of Rape in the South African Lowveld'. In *Men Behaving Differently? South African Men since 1994*, ed. Graeme Reid and Liz Walker, 65-88. Cape Town: Double Storey.

O'Meara, Dan. 1989. *Forty Lost Years: The Apartheid State and the Politics of the National Party, 1948-1994*. Athens, Ohio: Ohio University Press.

Padarath, Ashnie. 1998. 'Women and Violence in KwaZulu-Natal'. In *What Women Do in War Time: Gender and Conflict in Africa*, ed. Meredeth Turshen and Clotilde Twagiramariya. New York: Zed Books.

Palitza, Kristin. 2005. 'Abuse Survivors Still Waiting for Justice'. *Children FIRST* 59 (January/February 2005). Available at http://www.childrenfirst.org.za, accessed 20 January 2007.

Posel, Deborah. 2005a. ' "Baby Rape": Unmaking Secrets of Sexual Violence in Post-Apartheid South Africa'. In *Men Behaving Differently? South African Men since 1994*, ed. Graeme Reid and Liz Walker, 21-64. Cape Town: Double Storey.

———. 2005b. 'Sex, Death and the Fate of the Nation: Reflections on the Politicization of Sexuality in Post-Apartheid South Africa'. *Africa* 75(2): 125-53.

POWA (People Opposing Women Abuse). n.d. Statistics available at http://www.powa.co.za, accessed 12 February 2007.

Ramphele, Mamphela. 1993. *A Bed Called Home: Life in the Migrant Labour Hostels*. Athens, Ohio: Ohio University Press.

———. 2000. 'Teach Me How To Be a Man'. In *Violence and Subjectivity*, ed. V. Das, A. Kleinman, M. Ramphele and P. Reynolds. Berkeley: University of California Press.

Randera, Fazel. 2006. 'Bringing the Underground AIDS Fight to Surface'. *Creamer Media's Mining Weekly*. Available at http://www.miningweekly.co.za/min/views/columnist/hollard_R/, accessed 23 June 2006.

Reid, Graeme and Liz Walker (eds.). 2005. *Men Behaving Differently? South African Men since 1994*. Cape Town: Double Storey.

Renton, Alex. 2007. 'The Rape Epidemic'. *Observer Woman*, December: 50-56.

Reuters. 2006. 'Circumcision May Stop 1.4 mln HIV Cases in S. Africa'. Reuters report, 21 December. Available at http://www.alertnet.org/thenews/newsdesk/L21533533.htm, accessed 4 January 2008.

———. 2007. 'Group Hopes ANC Leader Promotes AIDS "Glasnost" '. Reuters report, 11 December. Available at http://www.africa.reuters.com/world/news/usnL11375416.html, accessed 9 January 2008.

SAPA (South African Press Association). 2007. 'Madlala-Routledge's Dismissal Slammed'. *Mail & Guardian* 9 August. Available at http://www.mg.co.za/articlePage.aspx?articleid=316175, accessed 9 January 2008.

Schoofs, Mark. 1999. 'All That Glitters (How HIV Caught Fire in South Africa – Part One: Sex and the Migrant Miner)'. *The Body: The Compact HIV/AIDS Resource* 28 April. Available at http://www.thebody.com/schoofs/glitters.html, accessed 22 June 2006.

Shisana, Olive and Leickness Simbayi. 2002. *Nelson Mandela HSRC Study of HIV/AIDS: Executive Summary South African National HIV Prevalence, Behavioural Risks and Mass Media. Household Survey 2002*. Cape Town: HSRC Press.

Spiegel, P. and H. Haroff-Tavel. 2006. 'HIV and Internally Displaced Persons, a Review of the Evidence'. Abstract CDE 0390, presented at the sixteenth International Aids Conference, held in Toronto, Canada, 13–18 August.

The Surplus People's Project. 1983a. *Forced Removals in South Africa* Vol. 1. Pietermaritzburg: The Surplus People's Project.

———. 1983b. *Forced Removals in South Africa* Vol. 5. Pietermaritzburg: The Surplus People's Project.

Turshen, Meredeth and Clotilde Twagiramariya (eds.). 1998. *What Women Do in War Time: Gender and Conflict in Africa*. New York: Zed Books.

UNAIDS (Joint United Nations Programme on HIV/AIDS). 2006. '2006 Report of the Global AIDS Epidemic: A UNAIDS 10th Anniversary Special Edition'. Geneva: UNAIDS. Available at http://www.data.unaids.org/pub/GlobalReport/2006/2006_GR-ExecutiveSummary_en.pdf, accessed 23 January 2007.

UNAIDS (Joint United Nations Programme on HIV/AIDS) and WHO (World Health Organisation). 2006a. 'Aids Epidemic Update'. Geneva: UNAIDS.

———. 2006b. 'Sub-Saharan Africa: Aids Epidemic Update'. Geneva: UNAIDS, December. Available at http://www.unaids.org/en/HIV_data/epi2006/, accessed 23 January 2007.

Vetten, Lisa and Kailash Bhana. 2001. *Violence, Vengeance and Gender: A Preliminary Investigation into the Links between Violence against Women and HIV/AIDS in South Africa*. Johannesburg and Cape Town: Centre for the Study of Violence and Reconciliation.

Whiteside, Alan and Clem Sunter. 2000. *AIDS: The Challenge for South Africa*. Cape Town: Human and Rousseau.

Wojcicki, Janet M. 2002. '"She Drank His Money": Survival Sex and the Problem of Violence in Taverns in Gauteng Province, South Africa'. *Medical Anthropology Quarterly* 16(3), September: 267–93.

Zwi, Anthony B. and A. Jorge Cabral. 1991. 'Identifying "High Risk Situations" for Preventing AIDS'. *British Medical Journal* 303: 1 527–529.

3

Human Rights in the Context of Human Security

•

Edwin Cameron and Marlise Richter[1]

Introduction

Department of Health (DoH) statistics show that from January to October 1989, 64 cases of HIV/AIDS were officially diagnosed in South Africa (Shisana and Zungu-Dirwayi 2003). Eighteen years later, there are more than five million South Africans living with the virus,[2] with an estimated 1 400 people infected every day (Venter 2006, 2–6). The virus has claimed millions of lives worldwide, but mostly in sub-Saharan Africa (UNAIDS and WHO 2005).

The devastation the epidemic brings often sparks calls for the curtailment of the human rights of people living with HIV/AIDS (PLWHA) and for a return to more traditional public health strategies, including mandatory testing, partner-tracking and official notification. However, since it began, with some notable exceptions, the South African AIDS epidemic has been approached from a pronounced human rights perspective. This can probably be traced to one of the ways in which internal opposition to apartheid was successful during the 1980s – by a broad legal attack proceeding from public interest and rights premises. The culture of human rights that persisted in resistance to apartheid came to fruition with the adoption of the Constitution in 1994, which renounced law as an instrument of oppression in favour of a framework of constitutional principles that promised human rights and the progressive realisation of human security for all.

These same human rights conceptions have underscored the national response to HIV/AIDS in South Africa. Starting with the strong criticism that the incipient HIV/AIDS policies of the National Party government faced in the 1980s and early

1990s, it was evident that human rights concerns would be foundational to HIV/ AIDS policy formulation in this country. It followed logically, then, that the National AIDS Convention of South Africa (NACOSA) plan adopted by the government of national unity in August 1994, enunciated – at least in principle – an unequivocal commitment to human rights. The advent of South Africa's Constitution – first the interim Constitution and, from 1997, the Constitution itself – created an enforceable human rights framework and the basis for a public discourse premised on human rights claims, including mechanisms to actualise rights to healthcare.

The debate about AIDS and how to deal with the epidemic could have been framed in a myriad of different ways: alternative approaches, based largely or solely on epidemiology, virology, public-health principles, or a politicised conception of race or gender, could have dominated the public discourse on HIV/AIDS. Yet, for the contingent reasons of history outlined above, the complex issues of transmission, stigma, testing, disclosure and access to treatment have been debated and constructed primarily in terms of human rights claims, entitlements and duties – and thus also in terms of human security. Even though South Africa's subcontinental neighbours have experienced epidemics of similar scale, it is this feature – the emphatic framing of issues of epidemiology in terms of human rights – that distinguishes South Africa from other African countries.

It was only a matter of time, therefore, before AIDS activists turned to the Constitution to frame and enforce their claims about how the government should respond to the epidemic. This chapter focuses specifically on subsection 27(1)(a) of the Bill of Rights of South Africa's Constitution, which provides that everyone has the right to have access to healthcare services and that the state must take reasonable legislative and other measures, within its available resources, to achieve the progressive realisation of this right (subsection 27(2)). The chapter illustrates how the right of access to treatment has been interpreted and enforced through the landmark legal action of the Treatment Action Campaign (TAC) against the Minister of Health in 2002, which sought to pressurise the South African government to provide accessible prophylactic antiretroviral (ARV) treatment for South African infants (see also Chapter 4 in this volume). Also discussed is how the 2002 decision in *Treatment Action Campaign v the Minister of Health* ('the TAC case')[3] illuminates the commitment of the judiciary and large parts of civil society to a human rights-based response to the epidemic, and how the case compelled the government to give substance to this right for pregnant women with HIV/AIDS.

Our chapter begins by providing a brief overview of different conceptions of human security and how these relate to the devastating impact that the HIV/AIDS epidemic has on people's lives. It then turns to the Constitutional Court's pronouncements in the TAC case and shows how this judgment challenged manifestations of AIDS denialism on the part of government leaders and played a vital role in shifting government policy on the roll-out of ARVs in the public sector.

Definitions of human security

It has rightly been pointed out that 'human security is an elastic and contested notion' (Acharya 2005). Former United Nations (UN) Secretary-General, Kofi Annan, describes human security thus:

> Human security in its broadest sense embraces far more than the absence of violent conflict. It encompasses human rights, good governance, access to education and health care and ensuring that each individual has opportunities and resources to fulfil his or her own potential. Every step in this direction is also a step towards reducing poverty, achieving economic growth and preventing conflict, [and towards] freedom from want, freedom from fear, and the freedom of future generations to inherit a healthy natural environment. (cited in Muloongo 2005, 1)

The term 'human security' was first used in a UN Development Programme (UNDP) Human Development Report (for more on this, see Chapter 1 in this volume), which described the concept as: 'safety for people from both violent and non-violent threats. It is a condition or state of being characterised by freedom from pervasive threats to people's rights, their safety, or even their lives.' (1994, 2)

Norman Mlambo observes that past notions of security in South Africa were generally narrow and primarily concerned with 'the security of the state against a perceived communist takeover' and 'keeping the communist threat at bay' (2005, 229). There has been a move away from narrow definitions based on wars, violent conflicts and communist or terrorist attacks, to a more holistic vision of security that embraces notions of individual well-being. It is particularly important that these broad notions of human security are applied in South Africa in order to measure and track the devastation wrought by the HIV/AIDS epidemic, as well as to assist in alleviating the epidemic's immediate and long-term consequences. Ramesh Thakur provides a useful definition of this broader concept of human security:

> Human security refers to the quality of life of the people of a society or polity. Anything which degrades their quality of life – democratic pressures, diminished access to or stock or resources, and so on – is a security threat. Conversely, anything which can upgrade their quality of life – economic growth, improved access to resources, social and political empowerment, and so on – is an enhancement of human security. (1997, 53–54)

Elhadj Sy argues that the basic elements that make up human security are survival, safety, opportunity, dignity, agency and autonomy (2001). The intimate connection between human security and human rights is plain – if the human rights of all people are respected and upheld, many of the requirements of human security are fulfilled. It follows that the illness, mortality, sense of stigma, discrimination, loss of income and support that are associated with the HIV/AIDS epidemic directly degrade human security – not only in the lives of PLWHA and their immediate families, but also for the broader public and the functioning of democracy itself (see Chirambo 2006). Any intervention that manages the physical manifestations of HIV/AIDS (in treating the virus and/or the opportunistic infections associated with it), prevents new infections, empowers PLWHA and upholds their dignity and freedom would thus directly enhance human security within the context of the epidemic.

Human security and the HIV/AIDS epidemic: Differentiating the human impact

In employing the concept of 'human' security, it is important not to overlook inherent gender dimensions. Heidi Hudson warns:

> Feminists . . . point out that an understanding of security issues needs to be extended to include the specific security concerns of women. There is a real danger that collapsing femininity or masculinity into the term 'human' could conceal the gendered underpinnings of security

practices. The term 'human' is presented as though it were gender-neutral, but very often it used an expression of the masculine. (2005, 157)

It is important to highlight women's experiences of HIV/AIDS when considering the human security implications of the epidemic. A substantial body of research has accumulated over the last fifteen years, which shows that women are particularly vulnerable to HIV/AIDS. Women are generally more at risk of contracting HIV for biological, social and economic reasons.[4] While treatment interventions, such as ARVs and research into female-controlled barrier methods, such as microbicides and the female condom, attempt to mitigate the biological impact of HIV/AIDS, the social and economic inequalities that women face require more complex enquiry and interventions. This is the result of an intricate interplay of social and political factors, of which the most pronounced is unequal power relations between men and women, which profoundly impact on women's ability to negotiate sex, and specifically safer sex (see, for example, Roa Gupta 2000, 18–20; Campbell, Mzaidume and Williams 1998, 50–58). The *World Disasters Report 2000* graphically describes this dangerous dynamic: 'More crucial . . . is [women's] economic dependence on men. AIDS raises questions of women's authority over their bodies. According to Milicent Obaso, a leading Kenyan authority on reproductive health, "most African women are unable to say 'no' to sex, even when they know they should, because to do so would threaten their security."' (ICRC 2001, 59)

Many women and girls face the threat of violence and abuse from their intimate male partners on a daily basis and many face additional abuse when they refuse sex or demand safer sex.[5] Economic dependence on men increases women's vulnerability to intimate partner violence (see Pendry 1998; Bhana et al. 2004; Jewkes et al. 1999), while a lack of education and employment opportunities can push women into sex work as their only means of survival (see UNAIDS 2002). Certain cultural practices such as virginity testing and wife inheritance also make women more vulnerable to contracting HIV (see Pieterse 2000; Richter 2004; Leclerc-Madala 2001, 2003; Albertyn 2003). All of these factors contribute to women's social position in society and increase their risk of HIV infection.

The impact of HIV/AIDS on human security

Lindy Heinecken draws a parallel between the 9/11 attacks in New York City in September 2001 and HIV/AIDS:

> The world reeled on 11 September 2001 as the United States (US) fell
> victim to the worst ever terrorist attack in history, killing over 3 000
> people. Yet in Africa, where a silent killer – HIV/AIDS – is sweeping
> through the continent killing an estimated 6 000 people a day, most
> remain mute. Few realise that this disease is as great, if not a greater,
> transnational security threat than terrorism. Already, more than ten
> times as many people are dying from AIDS than from wars in sub-
> Saharan Africa. (2001, 8)

Although it is open to debate whether the HIV/AIDS epidemic and terrorism pose
a threat comparable to traditional security concerns, the UN has identified HIV/
AIDS as a significant threat to stability and security. In 2000, the UN adopted
Resolution 1 308, which recognised the tremendous importance of HIV/AIDS 'given
its possible growing impact on social instability and emergency situations' (UNSC
2000). In 2001, the UN General Assembly Special Session on HIV/AIDS (UNGASS)
noted that the epidemic posed challenges in the armed forces, emergency situations,
as well as humanitarian disasters among others (see UN 2001; Lamboray 2002; see
also Chapter 11 in this volume).

Ulf Kristofferson argues that there are two core – and clearly interrelated –
dimensions to human security and HIV/AIDS: the challenge of human survival and
the threat to socio-economic development (2000). While features of the disease's
progression and the stigma still associated with it help to make AIDS a so-called
'silent killer', the death, morbidity and developmental implications of the epidemic
are anything but silent.

In their research on the impact of HIV/AIDS on human security, Pieter Fourie
and Martin Schönteich track the devastating impact of the epidemic on food security,
political stability, humanitarian emergencies, the armed forces and peacekeeping,
and levels of crime (2001, 2006). These and other issues are documented in the
other chapters of this book and although the early claims about the impact of the
epidemic on certain aspects of human security may have been exaggerated, the
adverse impact is indubitable. A few examples of the interplay of human security
and HIV/AIDS are noted below.

Hein Marais describes the far-reaching effects of HIV/AIDS on people's 'well-
being' (or human security) in the following way:

AIDS threatens well-being primarily along two tracks: by sapping the productivity of (and eventually killing) household members, and by imposing additional financial and labour needs. These effects and the responses they elicit usually are hitched into a standard sequence. Additional, sometimes extraordinary, care needs force trade-offs (for instance, withdrawing other household members from school or work in order to care for the ill). The ill person's income diminishes and his or her productive labour ebbs, and eventually disappears. Meanwhile, rising medical and related expenses (and, eventually, funeral and memorial costs) compel households to drain their savings, take on more debt and sell precious assets. (2005, 46)

Those elements that erode human security, such as poverty, lack of access to services and education, poor living conditions and unequal power relations, fuse to enhance the risk of contracting HIV, while the consequences of being HIV-positive further erode human security. Other consequences include an increase in labour costs,[6] wide-ranging effects on democracy and political processes (Manning 2002), an increase in the number of orphans and children requiring care,[7] as well as massive obstacles to reaching the Millennium Development Goals (MDGs) (O'Grady 2004; see also Chapter 10 in this volume).

Various studies have documented how the epidemic exacts a greater toll on women. Kristofferson writes: 'The security of women is particularly at risk. Whether it is economic security, food security, health security, personal or political security, women and girls are affected in a very specific way due to their physical, emotional and material differences and due to the important social, economic, and political inequalities existing between men and women.' (2000, 2) Because women are generally responsible for the care work in households and societies, having an ill person in the household increases directly the burden of support on women and girls (see, for example, Akintola 2006). Chronic illness also impacts on girls, who are sometimes withdrawn from school to help provide care (UNICEF 2005). As Marais points out, if the woman is ill herself, the consequences are even more severe:

Almost three quarters of 'AIDS-affected' households in South Africa are female-headed, a significant proportion of women are also battling

AIDS-related illnesses themselves.[8] The epidemic's impact therefore pivots especially on the ways in which women are being affected . . . [According to De Waal and Whiteside (2003):] '[Women's] burdens are greater, their time limited, and their lives shortened. Can social reproduction be secured when half of all adult women die before they are forty?' (Marais 2005, 53)

It is thus clear that while the HIV/AIDS epidemic threatens the human security of individuals, communities and countries as a whole, it is PLWHA, their immediate and extended families and women whose security is most threatened. It is for this reason that it is vital to differentiate the gendered impact of the epidemic. Moreover, in describing the extent of human security in South Africa, attention should be paid, for example, to:

- the extent to which post-exposure prophylaxis (PEP) against HIV infection is provided to rape survivors – who, overwhelmingly, are women;
- whether comprehensive prevention of mother-to-child transmission of HIV (PMTCT) programmes are available to all;
- the extent to which women with HIV/AIDS can exercise reproductive choices in line with their sexual and reproductive rights;
- the extent to which women can negotiate safer sex;
- how harmful cultural practices impact on the lives of women; and
- how the disproportionate burden of care that falls on the shoulders of women can be mitigated.

Looming over these stark material and physiological effects is the issue of stigma and its burden. Other diseases – notably tuberculosis – have been surrounded by stigma; but none so intractably and intensely as AIDS. Two factors serve to produce the acute stigma experienced by PLWA and their families: the fact that HIV/AIDS is sexually transmitted and that it is still preponderantly fatal in Africa, where ARV medication is not yet sufficiently available. The first of these remains as intractable as ever, clouding diagnosis and disclosure and impeding access to treatment, always more intensely in the case of women, who are often seen – incorrectly – as bearers of unwellness and contamination. The impact of the second factor – the seeming inevitability of death – is diminishing, as medical management of the virus has improved and governments have begun to distribute ARVs through their public health systems.

The external manifestations of stigma, most particularly discrimination and social ostracism, are well documented. What is less understood and studied are its internal dimensions: within the person living with HIV/AIDS, stigma saps well-being, confidence and dignity, impeding a sense of entitlement to, and thus accessing of, help, support and treatment.[9] Stigma is thus an important part of any assessment of the impact of the epidemic on human security, for it exacerbates the effects of HIV/AIDS and increases the load on those most affected by the virus.

The Treatment Action Campaign's PMTCT case
The right of access to healthcare

It is estimated that about 60 000 babies contracted HIV in South Africa in 1999 through mother-to-child transmission. If a national PMTCT programme had been in place, between one-sixth and one-third of these (between 19 595 and 23 105 babies) could have avoided infection with HIV (Geffen 2001; see also supporting affidavits by Dr Quarraisha Abdool Karim and Dr Robin Wood, filed in support of the TAC's 2001 case). The fact that ARV therapy was then not available in the public sector, meant that most, if not all of these infants died before their second birthdays. Despite the ample medical evidence to show that a short course of Zidovudine (AZT) or Nevirapine – both ARV drugs – would significantly reduce the risk of mother-to-child transmission, DoH policy prohibited medical facilities from providing these medicines to pregnant mothers with HIV/AIDS, unless directed by the Department. The DoH selected one urban and one rural site in each of South Africa's nine provinces to provide PMTCT, which were designated as PMTCT 'pilot sites'. Activists regarded the government's response as not only agonisingly slow, but as emblematic of its obstructive, denialist approach to both the causes of AIDS and its medical management (see Cameron 2003a, 2003b).

The TAC and other civil society organisations challenged the government's policy as unreasonable and claimed it was responsible for thousands of unnecessary and premature deaths.[10] The TAC initiated various forms of protest aimed at pressuring the government into extending the number of PMTCT sites. These included meetings, pickets, vigils, marches and petitions. When these activities were unsuccessful in changing the Department's policy, the TAC instituted legal action against the Minister of Health on 21 August 2001. The TAC and its co-applicants – who included Sarah

Hlalele, a mother who had herself lost the chance to save her baby from HIV because treatment was denied her – argued that the government's policy violated a number of human rights (for Sarah Hlalele's story, see Cameron (with Geffen) 2005, 201–03). These encompassed the right to access healthcare services, including subsection 27(1)(a), embracing 'reproductive health care' and the right of every child to basic healthcare services (in this case, the TAC referred to subsection 28(1)(c) of the Constitution, which stipulates the right to 'social security, including, if they are unable to support themselves and their dependants, appropriate social assistance').

The TAC won a favourable judgment in the High Court in December 2001, when Mr Justice Botha ordered the government to expand its PMTCT programme. When the government appealed this decision, the case was heard in the Constitutional Court (see the judgment of *TAC v Minister of Health* 2002 (4) BCLR 356 (T)). In July 2002, the Constitutional Court delivered a judgment in the applicants' favour. It ordered the government to extend its PMTCT programme beyond the pilot sites. In particular, the Court ordered that the government 'without delay' remove the restrictions that withheld Nevirapine from women with HIV/AIDS who wished to take the drug where it was medically indicated. It ordered the government to provide training for counsellors on the use of Nevirapine and to 'take reasonable measures to extend the testing and counselling facilities at hospitals and clinics throughout the public health sector' (*Minister of Health and Others v Treatment Action Campaign and Others* (2) 2002 (5) SA 721 at 765 at para. 135 E-H).

The Court drew the following connection between the provision of Nevirapine and a child's well-being or security:

> The provision of a single dose of Nevirapine to mother and child for the purpose of protecting the child against the transmission of HIV is, as far as the children are concerned, essential. Their needs are 'most urgent' and their inability to have access to Nevirapine profoundly affects their ability to enjoy all rights to which they are entitled. Their rights are 'most in peril' as a result of the policy that has been adopted and are most affected by a rigid and inflexible policy that excludes them from having access to Nevirapine. (*Minister of Health and Others v Treatment Action Campaign and Others* (2) 2002 (5) SA 721 at 765 at para. 78).

Access to adequate healthcare services and treatment is an elemental and indispensable component of a person's health, well-being and security. Medicines not only keep people alive and enable them to live productive and full lives and look after themselves and others, but they also prevent illness and death. The judgments of both the High Court and the Constitutional Court in the TAC case acknowledged this intimate relationship between healthcare and life. The Courts' orders in effect charged the state, within its means, to safeguard this particular component of human security, by making prophylactic ARV treatment available to pregnant women with HIV/AIDS. And indeed the provision of Nevirapine not only has directly life-saving properties for a baby – it also has a powerful and direct impact on the life and security of the mother. Because of its power and illustrative force, it is appropriate to quote at some length one of the deponents in the TAC case – 29-year-old Busisiwe Maqungo:

> I was tested for HIV in Conradie Hospital, Pinelands in May 1999, when my daughter, Nomazizi, then aged one month, was very sick. She suffered from various illnesses including pneumonia, diarrhoea and dehydration. Doctors decided to test her and the results came back positive. Automatically I went for the HIV test and tested positive. At that time I lived with the father of my baby in Langa. Since then my child was always in and out of hospital . . .
>
> I was hurt for my child when I found out that she was HIV-positive. I never suspected that I could be positive. The antenatal clinic that I visited before giving birth, never mentioned HIV. St Mary's antenatal clinic in Cape Town tested me during my pregnancy, but didn't tell me what it was for. I assumed that they had tested me for HIV as well. I saw that my file said something about being positive, but the nurse said it had something to do with iron, which I didn't understand . . .
>
> I gave birth to an HIV-positive child and wondered why, if she could be saved with AZT. I should have been told what I was tested for and asked if I wanted to be tested for HIV. If there was a program in all hospitals where mothers book and women were asked to be tested for HIV, I would have gone for a test. And if doctors had given me information about treatment to prevent my baby from getting HIV, I would have tried to get it, for the sake of my baby . . .

> I breastfed my baby for two weeks then she stopped. I had to buy formula milk for her which cost R24 for a 500g tin. A tin could last up to two weeks if I fed my child with other food like vegetables as well. Only after my child was diagnosed and she had lost considerable weight was I able to get formula milk from Conradie Hospital . . .
>
> My baby was always sick. I had to borrow money from her father's parents, to take her to hospital. She normally had to go to Red Cross or Conradie Hospital and she was once admitted in Tygerberg Hospital. Sometimes my baby would be out of hospital for a week and then she would be sick again. I never had enough time with her . . .
>
> Doctors always told me that my baby will die and that there was nothing they could do for her. I knew my baby would die, but I didn't want to hear it, especially not from the doctors all the time. My baby received no special medicines after she was diagnosed, she got the same medicines normally given to HIV-negative children . . .
>
> The government should give people with HIV anti-retroviral drugs because they need it. The government should implement PMTCT nationally so that women can be given a choice and their children can be saved. People with HIV should also get treatment for opportunistic infections . . . (TAC 2001)

This account poignantly and vividly shows how Busisiwe would have been spared anguish, despair and heartbreak if she had received adequate and sensitive healthcare and had she been given the choice of taking Nevirapine to reduce the risk of transmitting HIV to Nomazizi. A child who was HIV-negative would have saved the money, care and resources (to speak only materially) that Busisiwe was forced to invest in Nomazizi's health – expenses that most likely occurred at some financial cost to her, as well as costs to her own health and security.[11] This case illustrates the explicit link between the government's response to the epidemic and direct human security concerns. It illustrates the direct impact of HIV on human security and shows what a rights-based approach can achieve through well-targeted public interest advocacy and litigation.

The implications of AIDS denialism for human security
The TAC case was decided at a time when South Africa's response to HIV/AIDS was marred by the government's persistent reluctance to accept unequivocally and

publicly that HIV causes AIDS.[12] This 'AIDS denialism'[13] and its associated tenets, such as that ARVs were toxic, HIV testing was of uncertain benefit and descriptions of the South African AIDS epidemic as 'explosive' were inaccurate, underlay the government's chief arguments before the Constitutional Court.[14] The Court's judgment sent a strong message warning against delays in preventing HIV infections and against inhibiting people's right to choose to receive ARVs. While this decision dealt with a limited issue – the availability of a single-dose or short course of treatment to a pregnant mother with HIV for purely prophylactic reasons – it foreshadowed more comprehensive moves by the Courts to ensure that PLWHA have access to treatment. The judgment became a powerful instrument in the hands of civil society, not only because of the practical impact of the order it embodied, but also because of its tone and its affirmation of rational scientific understandings of the epidemic and it formed the foundation for further government deliberation on providing broader access to treatment of PLWHA.

The effects of the judgment were soon felt. The Constitutional Court handed down its judgment on 5 July 2002. Thirteen months later, on 8 August 2003, and nearly four anguished years after denialism first manifested itself in executive statements, the government at last announced 'its principled approach that antiretroviral drugs do help improve the quality of life of those at a certain stage of the development of AIDS, if administered properly' and charged the DoH with developing a comprehensive plan on universal treatment (Special Cabinet Meeting Statement 2003). Over a month later, the government committed itself to the 'Operational Plan for Comprehensive Treatment and Care for HIV and AIDS' and to distributing ARVs through the public health system (see Minister of Health 2003).

Looking to the future

The AIDS epidemic graphically underscores the vulnerability of many impoverished Africans to disease and its burdens. It also draws attention to indefensible inequalities and distortions in the availability and distribution of essential medicines in resource-poor areas of the world, particularly sub-Saharan Africa (see Cameron and Berger 2005). Not only within South Africa, but globally, the TAC court case and the issues involved rightly attracted enormous attention, and the judgment, public acclaim. It focused the world's attention on AIDS in Africa (albeit not enduringly enough) and highlighted the stark inequalities between access to treatment in 'developed' countries and the lack of treatment in 'developing' countries. The critical question is whether the momentum that the case generated can be sustained.

Following the Constitutional Court judgment, the TAC and other activist organisations took a lead in monitoring the roll-out and quality of the government's PMTCT programme. The 2003 *South African Health Review* reported that, following the TAC case, there has been 'a gradual and steady expansion of the PMTCT programme beyond the original pilot sites' (see Doherty et al. 2003, 5). In 2004, Rob Dorrington et al. found that the proportion of facilities providing PMTCT increased from 20 per cent in 2002 to 53 per cent in 2003, but they could not obtain information on the number of mothers who have received treatment, nor on the impact that it is having (2004, 1). For at least three years, there were no official reports explaining progress in the roll-out of PMTCT.[15] However, in March 2006, the DoH reported to UNGASS that 'an estimated 55 per cent of pregnant HIV-positive women received Nevirapine to reduce the risk of mother-to-child transmission (y) in public sector facilities in 2004' (2006c, 24). Worryingly, an earlier version of the report, dated February 2006, stated that 'using available PMTCT data on the NPBI-4 formula, an estimated 78.7 per cent of pregnant HIV-positive women received Nevirapine to reduce the risk of MTCT in public sector facilities in 2004' (DoH 2006b, 21).

These sometimes confusing versions of facts suggest that clear measurements of progress are hard to come by.[16] Furthermore, the possibility that almost half of pregnant women with HIV/AIDS had no access to a simple medical intervention that reduces HIV infection, four years after the programme was rolled out in 2001, is immensely distressing.

A shift in focus by both the government and civil society to the roll-out of universal treatment may have diverted attention away from the PMTCT programme. Yet it is vital that the momentum that the litigation generated be sustained, so that the programme becomes available to all women who need it, in order to prevent new infections. Mark Heywood makes this observation about the implementation of socio-economic rights (and thus also guarantees of human security) in relation to a number of other cases that touch on these issues:

> But, learning from the sequels to *Grootboom*, *Ngxuza (Permanent Secretary, Department of Welfare, Eastern Cape Provincial Government and Another v Ngxuza and Others* 2001 (4) SA 1184 and 2001 (10) BCLR 1039 (SCA) and other cases, there is an understanding that there will be shades and speeds of compliance by government with court orders concerning

socio-economic rights. This may range from active and vigorous implementation, to turgid and tortoise-like. (2003a, 3)

Furthermore, there is an understanding that – to a large extent – the pace will be dictated by the ongoing engagement of civil society organisations, including the Human Rights Commission (HRC), with the implementation of the Court's orders.

Overall, the government's response to HIV/AIDS has revealed a lamentable absence of impelling and overriding urgency. As Pierre de Vos points out: 'What has been lacking in the state's conduct is the sense of urgency, a sense that this is a life-and-death situation that requires immediate and drastic measures' (2003, 111). In early 2007, heartening signs of a new approach on the part of government – led by two women, Deputy-President Mlambo-Ngcuka and Deputy-Minister of Health Madlala-Routledge[17] – encouraged optimism that the foot-dragging may be ending. Yet it is vital that civil society reminds government, officials and healthcare workers at every opportunity of the urgency that the AIDS epidemic commands of us. Civil society needs to ensure that the government continues to implement the TAC case judgment, that the PMTCT programme progressively expands in order to become a viable option for all pregnant women with HIV/AIDS and that the programme is constantly updated in line with international best practice in order to ensure that the most efficacious and cost-effective medicines and procedures are made available to women.[18] At the same time, government promises made on universal roll-out need to be vigilantly monitored.[19] In particular, care should be taken to refer women who enter the healthcare system to receive antenatal care to the PMTCT programme and appropriate facilities, so that they can initiate ARVs when medically appropriate.

Conclusion

HIV/AIDS has dramatically diminished human security in South Africa. It has burdened the vulnerable and the poor, and exacerbated the deficiencies in their material living conditions. The stigma associated with infection with HIV and illness with AIDS increases these effects. However, the future offers considerable hope, provided that sufficient commitment exists at community, corporate and governmental levels. The provision of ARVs through the public healthcare system – whether for treatment or for preventative purposes – is essential for the successful management of the HIV/AIDS epidemic in South Africa. Access to adequate healthcare, treatment and prevention are vital components, not only for the human security of individuals, but also for the security and future of the nation as a whole.

Notes

1. We are grateful to the editors of this volume and to the anonymous reviewers for their helpful comments.
2. The most recent antenatal survey (DoH 2006a) estimates that that between 5.7 and 6.2 million people were living with HIV in 2004.
3. See *Treatment Action Campaign and Others v Minister of Health and Others* 2002 (4) SA BCLR 356, (T); *Minister of Health and Others v Treatment Action Campaign and Others* 2002 (5) SA 717 (CC) and *Minister of Health v Treatment Action Campaign* (No. 2) 2002 (5) SA 721 (CC).
4. UNAIDS notes that women are two to four times more likely to contract HIV from unprotected vaginal intercourse than men. The reason for this is that: 'As compared to men, women have a bigger surface area of mucosa exposed during intercourse to their partner's sexual secretions (in women, the genital mucosa is the thin lining of the vagina and cervix). Semen infected with HIV typically contains a higher concentration of virus than a woman's sexual secretions. This makes male-to-female transmission more efficient than female-to-male.' (UNAIDS 1997, 3; see also Greenblatt and Hessol 2000).
5. Marais argues,
    > Research is also confirming a strong association between sexual and other forms of abuse against women, which increases the odds of becoming HIV-infected. The links between intimate partner violence and an increased likelihood of HIV infection, for example, appear solid. At antenatal clinics in Soweto, HIV infection was found to be significantly more common in women who had been physically abused by their partners than in those who had not been abused. (2005, 46)
6. According to the *World Disasters Report 2000*, GDP in most countries in sub-Saharan Africa will have declined by at least 14 per cent and per capita income by 10 per cent by 2005 because of AIDS, if the UN analysis is accurate. Morbidity and absenteeism cause an increase in the cost of labour, which means that companies are more likely to automate production, as is already happening in South Africa. This is more expensive, but saves companies from the cost and time of constantly training new employees (ICRC 2001).
7. More than 1 700 children are infected with HIV daily, while HIV/AIDS is more likely than any other cause of death to produce double orphans (UNAIDS 2004, 11, 14; Gosh and Kalipeni 2004).
8. Marais (2005) refers here to the study by Steinberg et al. (2002).
9. The internal dimension of stigma and self-disentitlement is discussed in Cameron (with Geffen 2005).
10. The applicants in the case were the TAC, Dr Haroon Saloojee and the Children's Rights Centre. When the case reached the Constitutional Court, the Community Law Centre, the Institute for Democracy in South Africa (IDASA) and Cotlands Baby Sanctuary joined as *amicus curia* (friends of the court) in support of the applicants' arguments. Notably the Human Rights Commission and the Commission for Gender Equality did not intervene, despite that fact that the case clearly constituted a human rights, as well as a women's rights issue.
11. For an excellent analysis of the economic costs and benefits of a PMTCT programme, see Nattrass (2003).

12. For an account of the history of the South African government's engagement with the epidemic in the last fifteen years, see Shisana and Zungu-Dirwayi (2003) and MacFarlane (2004). According to Marais:

> Questioning and critiquing the accuracy of information and dominant understandings of HIV/AIDS have served as a prelude not for refining and acting on that knowledge but for denying the epidemic's very existence. This should not surprise us. For the rhetoric and sensibilities that have evolved into the 'denialism' associated with President Mbeki and others in the African National Congress government are only nominally about AIDS, science and poverty. To a considerable extent, 'denialism' functions as a grammar for other, overarching political engagements and pursuits. And AIDS serves such an enterprise not as a mere pretext, but because it draws into focus so many outrages and injustices. (2005, 18)

13. Recently, terminological questions have been raised about whether it is most appropriate to brand President Mbeki's scepticism about the aetiology of AIDS 'denialism', 'dissidence' or 'scepticism'. The terminology is irrelevant to the substantive point at issue.

14. For a discussion of the politics and controversies surrounding the case, see Heywood (2003b). For a discussion of the AIDS denialism arguments in the TAC case, as well as a comprehensive overview of AIDS denialism in South Africa, see Nattrass (2007).

15. The 2004 and 2005 South African National Health Reviews did not cover the PMTCT programmes.

16. Meyers et al. note, 'In 2002, South Africa set a goal to reduce the proportion of infants infected with HIV by 20 per cent by 2005. There is no reliable information to assess whether this has been achieved.' (2007, S475)

17. Regrettably, President Mbeki fired the Deputy-Minister of Health on 8 August 2007, on account of an unauthorised trip to Spain for an AIDS conference and her 'inability to work as part of a collective' (Mbeki 2007). Many believe that she was fired because of her outspoken views on HIV/AIDS that contradicted those of the president and because of her being candid about government department inefficiencies (see, for example, *Mail & Guardian* Reporter 2007).

18. Towards the end of 2007, the TAC urged government to urgently improve South Africa's lagging PMTCT programme. In particular, TAC noted four crucial points: '(1) increasing take-up of the programme, (2) upgrading the single-dose Nevirapine regimen, (3) ensuring women with low CD4 counts or AIDS are placed on highly active antiretroviral treatment (HAART) and (4) appropriately monitoring and evaluating the programme on a regular basis.' (2007)

19. Heywood writes:

> The disruption of livelihoods, and the diversion of scarce resources to fill gaps left by those who have died, will rob the millions of poor people of prospects for income accumulation and social improvement. It is in this context that the next challenge of the AIDS epidemic must be viewed – expanding access to treatment is not only a moral, medical and legal necessity – it is also one of the critical ways of addressing the development goals of South Africa. (2005, 382)

References

Acharya, Amitav. 2005. 'Human Security, Identity Politics and Global Governance: From Freedom from Fear to Fear of Freedoms'. Paper given at the international conference on 'Civil Society, Religion and Global Governance: Paradigms of Power & Persuasion', 1–2 September 2005, Canberra.

Akintola, Olagoke. 2006. 'Gendered Home-Based Care in South Africa: More Trouble for the Troubled'. *African Journal of AIDS Research* 5(3): 237–47.

Albertyn, Cathi. 2003. 'Contesting Democracy: HIV/AIDS and the Achievement of Gender Equality in South Africa'. *Feminist Studies* 29(3) (Fall): 595–615.

Bhana, Kailash, Liesl Gerntholtz, Karen Hurt, Andrea Meeson and Lisa Vetten. 2004. 'Health and Hope in Our Hands: Addressing HIV and AIDS in the Aftermath of Rape and Woman Abuse'. Johannesburg: AIDS Law Project, Centre for the Study of Violence and Reconciliation, Council for Scientific and Industrial Research and Jacana.

Cameron, Edwin. 2003a. 'Law in the Struggle for Truth'. *South African Law Journal* 120: 1–7.

———. 2003b. 'AIDS Denial and Holocaust Denial: AIDS, Justice and the Courts in South Africa'. *South African Law Journal I* 120: 525–39.

Cameron, Edwin (with Nathan Geffen). 2005. *Witness to AIDS*. Cape Town: Tafelberg/NB Publishers.

Cameron, Edwin and Jonathan Berger. 2005. 'Patents and Public Health: Principle, Politics and Paradox'. *Proceedings of the British Academy* 13: 331–69. Also published in David Vaver (ed.). 2005. *Intellectual Property Rights*. London: Routledge.

Campbell, Cathy, Yodwa Mzaidume and Brian Williams. 1998. 'Gender as an Obstacle to Condom Use: HIV Prevention amongst Commercial Sex Workers in a Mining Community'. *Agenda* 39: 50–58.

Chirambo, Kondwani. 2006. *Democratisation in the Age of AIDS – Understanding the Political Implications*. Cape Town: IDASA.

De Vos, Pierre. 2003. 'So Much to Do, So Little Done: The Right of Access to Anti-retroviral Drugs Post-Grootboom'. *Law, Democracy and Development* 7(1): 83–111.

De Waal, Alex and Alan Whiteside. 2003. 'New Variant Famine: AIDS and Food Crisis in Southern Africa'. *The Lancet* 362: 1 234–237.

DoH (Department of Health). 2006a. *National HIV and Syphilis Antenatal Sero-Prevalance Survey in South African in 2005*. Pretoria: DoH.

———. 2006b. *Progress Report on the Declaration of Commitment on HIV and AIDS*. Prepared for the United National General Assembly Special Session on HIV and AIDS (UNGASS), February.

———. 2006c. *Progress Report on the Declaration of Commitment on HIV and AIDS*. Prepared for the United National General Assembly Special Session on HIV and AIDS (UNGASS), March. Available at http://www.data.unaids.org/pub/Report/2006/2006_country_progress_report_south_africa_en.pdf, accessed 7 December 2006.

Doherty, Tanya, Mitchell Besser, Steven Donohue, Nelson Kamoga, Norah Stoops, Louisa Williamson and Ronel Visser. 2003. *Case Study Report on Implementation and Expansion of the PMTCT Programme in the Nine Provinces of South Africa*, Report (October). Durban: Health Systems Trust; Pretoria: Department of Health.

Dorrington, Rob, Debbie Bradshaw, Leigh Johnson and Debbie Budlender. 2004. *The Demographic Impact of HIV/AIDS in South Africa – National Indicators for 2004*. Cape Town: Centre for Actuarial Research, South African Medical Research Council and Actuarial Society of South Africa.

Fourie, Pieter and Martin Schönteich. 2001. 'Africa's New Security Threat: HIV/AIDS and Human Security in Africa'. *African Security Review* 10(4): 29–42.

———. 2006. 'Die, the Beloved Countries: Human Security and HIV/AIDS in Africa'. *Politeia* 21(2): 6–30. Available at http://www.sarpn.org.za/documents/d0000177/P170_Security_HIVAIDS. pdf, accessed 17 December 2007.

Geffen, Nathan. 2001. 'Cost and Cost-Effectiveness of Mother-to-Child Transmission Prevention of HIV'. Treatment Action Campaign Briefing Paper, 15 August. Available at http://www.tac.org.za/Documents/MTCTPrevention/mtctcost.rtf, accessed 7 December 2006.

Gosh, Jayati and Ezekiel Kalipeni. 2004. 'Rising Tide of AIDS Orphans in Southern Africa'. In *HIV/AIDS in Africa: Beyond Epidemiology*, ed. Ezekiel Kalipeni, Susan Craddock, Joseph R. Oppong and Jayati Ghosh, 305–15. Oxford: Blackwell Publishing.

Greenblatt, Ruth and Nancy Hessol. 2000. 'Epidemiology and Natural History of HIV Infection in Women'. In *A Guide to the Clinical Care of Women with HIV*, US Department of Human and Health Sciences, Health Resources and Services Administration, HIV/AIDS Bureau. Available at http://www.reproline.jhu.edu/video/hiv/tutorials/English/tutorials/HIV_overview/references/docs/epi_nh_guide.pdf, accessed 15 December 2006.

Hamilton, Georgina. 1998. 'Virgin Testing: One Answer to the AIDS Epidemic?' *Indicator SA* 15(3): 62–66.

Heinecken, Lindy. 2001. 'Living in Terror: The Looming Threat to Southern Africa'. *African Security Review* 10(4): 8–17.

Heywood, Mark. 2003a. 'Contempt or Compliance? The TAC Case after the Constitutional Court Judgment'. *ESR Review* 4(1) (March): 7–10.

———. 2003b. 'Preventing Mother-to-Child HIV Transmission in South Africa: Background, Strategies and Outcomes of the Treatment Action Campaign Case against the Minister of Health'. *South African Journal of Human Rights* 19(2): 278–315.

———. 2005. 'The Achilles Heel? The Impact of HIV/AIDS on Democracy in South Africa'. In *HIV/AIDS in South Africa*, ed. Salim Abdool Karim and Quarraisha Abdool Karim. Cambridge: Cambridge University Press.

Hudson, Heidi. 2005. '"Doing" Security as though Humans Matter: A Feminist Perspective on Gender and the Politics of Human Security'. *Security Dialogue* 36(2) (June): 155–74.

ICRC (International Federation of Red Cross and Red Crescent Societies). 2001. *World Disasters Report 2000 – Focus on Public Health*. Geneva: ICRC.

Jewkes, Rachel, Loveday Penn-Kekana, Jonathan Levin, Matsie Ratsaka and Margaret Schrieber. 1999. *'He Must Give Me Money, He Mustn't Beat Me': Violence against Women in Three South African Provinces*. Report. Pretoria: MRC (Medical Research Council).

Kristofferson, Ulf. 2000. 'HIV/AIDS as a Human Security Issue: A Gender Perspective'. Paper presented at the Expert Group Meeting on the HIV/AIDS Pandemic and its Gender Implications. 13–17 November in Windhoek. Available at http://www.un.org/womenwatch/daw/csw/hivaids/kristofferson.htm, accessed 11 December 2006.

Lamboray, Jean-Louis. 2002. 'HIV/AIDS and Security'. Paper presented at the WHO Consultation on Health and Human Security by the UNAIDS Chief of Technical Network Development 15-17 April in Cairo. Available at http://www.data.unaids.org/Topics/Security/Cairo_intervention_en.doc, accessed 15 December 2006.

Leclerc-Madala, Suzanne. 2001. 'Virginity Testing: Managing Sexuality in a Maturing HIV/AIDS Epidemic'. *Medical Anthropology Quarterly* 15(4): 533-52.

———. 2003. 'Protecting Girlhood? Virginity Revivals in the Era of AIDS'. *Agenda* 56: 16-25.

MacFarlane, Marco. 2004. 'HIV/AIDS: "The Most Devastating Health Crisis in History"'. *Fast Facts*. South African Institute of Race Relations 12 (December).

Mail & Guardian Reporter. 2007. 'Madlala-Routledge Was Set up'. *Mail & Guardian* 10 August. Available at http://www.mg.co.za/articlePage.aspx?articleid=316236&area=/insight/insight__national, accessed 30 November 2007.

Manning, Ryan. 2002. 'AIDS and Democracy: What Do We Know? A Literature Review'. Discussion paper prepared for the AIDS and Democracy: Setting the Research Agenda Workshop, 22-23 April. Cape Town: HEARD and IDASA. Available at http://www.ukzn.ac.za/heard/research/ResearchReports/2002/LiteratureReview.pdf, accessed 11 December 2006.

Marais, Hein. 2005. *Buckling: The Impact of AIDS in South Africa 2005*. Pretoria: University of Pretoria.

Mbeki, Thabo. 2007. 'Letter from the President'. ANC Today 7(32), 17-23 August. Available at http://www.anc.org.za/ancdocs/anctoday/2007/at32.htm, accessed 30 November 2007.

Meyers, Tammy, Harry Moultrie, Kimesh Naidoo, Mark Cotton, Brian Eley and Gayle Sherman. 2007. 'Challenges to Pediatric HIV Care and Treatment in South Africa'. *The Journal of Infectious Diseases* 196: S474-81.

Minister of Health, Dr Manto Tshabala-Msimang. 2003. 'Statement of Cabinet on a Plan for Comprehensive Treatment and Care for HIV and AIDS in South Africa', 19 November. Available at http://www.info.gov.za/speeches/2003/03111916531001.htm, accessed 7 December 2006.

Mlambo, Norman. 2005. 'Perceptions of Human Security in Democratic South Africa – Opinions of Students from Tertiary Institutions'. In *The Many Faces of Human Security – Case Studies of Seven Countries in Southern Africa*, ed. Keith Muloongo, Roger Kibasomba and Jemima Njeri Kariri. Pretoria: Institute of Security Studies.

Muloongo, Keith. 2005. 'Introduction'. In *The Many Faces of Human Security – Case Studies of Seven Countries in Southern Africa*, ed. Keith Muloongo, Roger Kibasomba and Jemima Njeri Kariri. Pretoria: Institute of Security Studies.

Muloongo, Keith, Roger Kibasomba and Jemima Njeri Kariri (eds.). *The Many Faces of Human Security – Case Studies of Seven Countries in Southern Africa*. Pretoria: Institute of Security Studies.

Nattrass, Nicoli. 2003. *The Moral Economy of AIDS*. Cambridge: Cambridge University Press.

———. 2007. *Mortal Combat – AIDS Denialism and the Struggle for Antiretrovirals in South Africa*. Pietermaritzburg: University of KwaZulu-Natal Press.

O'Grady, Mary. 2004. 'The Impoverishing Pandemic: The Impact of the HIV/AIDS Crisis in Southern Africa on Development'. *From Disaster to Development: HIV/AIDS in Southern Africa, Development Update* 5(3) (December): 17-44.

Pendry, Betsi. 1998. 'The Links between Gender Violence and HIV/AIDS'. *Agenda* 39: 30-33.

Pieterse, Marius. 2000. 'Beyond the Reach of Law? HIV, African Culture and Customary Law'. *Tydskrif vir die Suid-Afrikaanse Reg* 3: 428–44.

Richter, Marlise. 2004. 'Customary Law, Gender and HIV/AIDS'. *Gender Research Programme Bulletin* 1: 4–5.

Roa Gupta, Geeta. 2000. 'Gender, Sexuality, and HIV/AIDS: The What, the Why and the How'. *Women's Health Project Newsletter* 36 (November): 18–20.

Shisana, Olive and Zungu-Dirwayi, Nompumelelo. 2003. 'Government's Changing Response to HIV/AIDS'. *The Real State of the Nation – South Africa after 1990, Development Update Special Edition* 4(31) November: 165–87.

Special Cabinet Meeting Statement. 2003. 'Enhanced Programme against HIV and AIDS'. 8 August. Available at http://www.gcis.gov.za/media/cabinet/030808.htm, accessed 11 December 2006.

Steinberg, Malcolm, Saul Johnson, Gill Schierhout and David Ndegwa. 2002. *Hitting Home: How Households Cope with the Impact of the HIV/AIDS Epidemic*. Washington, DC: Henry J. Kaiser Foundation.

Sy, Elhadj. 2001. 'Gender, HIV/AIDS and Human Security'. Paper presented at the United Nations Commission on the Status of Women, 45th Session, 16 June. Available at http://www.un.org/womenwatch/daw/csw/Sy2001.htm, accessed 7 December 2006.

TAC (Treatment Action Campaign). 2001. 'Mother-to-Child Transmission Prevention Court Case Affidavits'. Available at http://www.tac.org.za/Documents/MTCTCourtCase/MTCTCourtCase.htm, accessed 19 June 2005.

———. 2007. 'Key World AIDS Day Message: We Must Improve Maternal Health and the Prevention of Mother-to-Child HIV Transmission Programme'. Electronic newsletter, available at http://www.tac.org.za/news_2007.html, accessed 30 November 2007.

Thakur, Ramesh. 1997. 'From National to Human Security'. In *Asia-Pacific Security: The Economics-Politics Nexus*, ed. Stuart Harris and Andrew Mack. Sydney: Allen and Unwin.

UN (United Nations). 2001. 'Declaration of Commitment on HIV/AIDS'. United Nations A/RES/S-26/2, 8th Plenary Meeting, 27 June.

UNAIDS (Joint United Nations Programme on HIV/AIDS). 1997. 'Women and AIDS'. *UNAIDS Best Practice Collection*. New York and Geneva: UNAIDS.

———. 2002. 'Sex Work and HIV/AIDS'. In *UNAIDS Technical Update* (June). New York and Geneva: UNAIDS.

———. 2004. *Children on the Brink 2004: A Joint Report of New Orphan Estimates and a Framework for Action*. New York: UNAIDS, UNICEF and USAID.

UNAIDS (Joint United Nations Programme on HIV/AIDS) and WHO (World Health Organisation). 2005. 'AIDS Epidemic Update: 2005'. New York and Geneva: UNAIDS and WHO.

UNDP (United Nations Development Programme). 1994. *New Developments in Human Security*. Human Development Report. Available at http://www.hdr.undp.org/en/reports/global/hdr1994/, accessed 23 March 2008.

UNICEF (United Nations (International) Children's (Emergency) Fund). 2005. *Gender Achievements and Prospects in Education. The GAP Report: Part One*. New York: UNICEF. Available at http://www.unicef.org/publications/files/GAP_Report_part1_final_14_Nov.pdf, accessed 15 December 2007.

UNSC (United Nations Security Council). 2000. 'UNSC Resolution 1308, on the Responsibility of the Security Council in the Maintenance of International Peace and Security: HIV/AIDS and International Peace-keeping Operations'. Adopted by the Security Council at its 4 172nd meeting, 17 July 2000.

Venter, Francois. 2006. 'The South African National Antiretroviral Programme: Is it on Track?' *AIDS Analysis Africa Online* Jan/Feb. Available at http://www.unisa.ac.za/contents/publications/docs/Polit212.pdf, accessed 7 December 2006.

4

The Treatment Action Campaign's Activism

Dean Peacock, Thokozile Budaza and Alan Greig

Introduction

Launched on International Human Rights Day on 10 December 1998, South Africa's Treatment Action Campaign (TAC) has demonstrated its ability to win major gains for people living with HIV/AIDS (PLWHA). Whether it is challenging the government to deliver on its constitutional commitments to the provision of adequate health services, supporting a prisoners' strike for access to antiretrovirals (ARVs) in Durban (Khan 2005), or mobilising thousands of high-school students in the Eastern Cape to march for better prevention strategies on the thirtieth anniversary of the Soweto youth uprising (TAC 2006), the TAC continues to be a critical voice of dissent.

A key characteristic of the TAC's activities has been its readiness and capacity to change its approach in response to the conditions and challenges it faces. This chapter investigates this ability to change by describing the TAC's attempt to shift from a relatively exclusive focus on treatment access to a strong focus on addressing the gender inequalities driving the spread and impact of the epidemic. Drawing on the growing literature on gender and HIV/AIDS, as well as on interviews with TAC activists, this chapter explores the TAC's work to challenge gender-based violence and to chart new forms of feminism that some within the organisation are calling 'AIDS feminism'. In doing so, this chapter profiles the TAC's campaign in Khayelitsha, in Cape Town, to bring to justice the murderers of the TAC activist, Lorna Mlofana, and concludes by reflecting on the implications and lessons learned from the TAC's efforts to address gender inequalities and gender-based violence.

The TAC and HIV/AIDS

The TAC arose as a response to the devastation being wrought by the HIV/AIDS epidemic in South Africa and the failure of the government to recognise and respond to the severity of the crisis. In April 2001, the TAC's campaigns for access to affordable medication led to unprecedented shifts in policy from the International Pharmaceutical Manufacturers' Association and to dramatic reductions in the prices of AIDS medications. A year later in July 2002, the TAC won a Constitutional Court case that obligated the government to put in place a national programme for the prevention of mother-to-child transmission (PMTCT). Sixteen months later, in November 2003, the South African government yielded to the TAC's demands and sustained civil disobedience campaigns, and announced the 'Operational Plan for Comprehensive HIV and AIDS Care, Management and Treatment for South Africa', which included commitments to make ARV therapy available across the country (DoH 2003).

When the South African government committed itself to a national ARV roll-out plan in November 2003, the TAC put its weight behind the successful implementation of all interventions aimed at alleviating the HIV/AIDS epidemic. At the 2005 TAC National Congress, Zackie Achmat, then the TAC chairperson, reflected on what this meant for the organisation, saying:

> [The] TAC's response recognised that the battle had shifted from the need for a national policy and programme to its implementation countrywide. Prior to the government's change in policy and programme, most of TAC's mobilising efforts were directed at national government, drug companies, and policy issues. The rollout meant that now every effort had to shift to ensure that programmes were implemented, and this was particularly important in provinces such as the Eastern Cape, KwaZulu-Natal, Limpopo and Mpumalanga. (TAC 2005)

To support the building of community capacity for support and holding the government accountable, the organisation has grown dramatically and expanded its focus. As of March 2007, the TAC's numbers have swelled to between 16 000 and 20 000 people[1] and the organisation has developed provincial offices in six of the nine provinces and in nine districts, with over 200 branches operating across the country. Its membership is overwhelmingly made up of people living with, or affected by HIV/AIDS and is based mostly in South Africa's townships and informal settlements.

The TAC's campaigns and activism are grounded in ongoing, widespread community-level work to promote treatment literacy among TAC activists and in their communities, so that community members understand that health, HIV and AIDS and medical treatment cannot be divorced from the political context in which they exist, and so that they can use new information to improve their lives and their communities (TAC 2005).

This focus has been little documented and discussed. Journalists have typically had a relatively narrow focus, chronicling the TAC's legal battles and its efforts to hold the government accountable, or writing about its senior leadership. More academic works have explored the organisation's origins in the anti-apartheid and gay rights movements of the 1980s and 1990s (see, for example, Mbali 2005), described its organisational philosophy and relationship to social movements and the South African government (Friedman and Mottiar 2005; De Waal 2006), documented the TAC's use of rights-based activism to secure critical health services (Annas 2003, 750–54), and chronicled the development of political identities among TAC activists (see, for example, Robins 2004; Mosoetsa 2005). But to date, little has been written about the TAC's work at community level. As Zackie Achmat put it in a speech at the 2005 TAC Congress in Cape Town:

> Few [TAC] sympathisers know much about the nature and extent of its grassroots work . . . The TAC that few people see or understand is an army of 10 000 members and volunteers across the country, working continuously in their communities to educate people about HIV and their own health on a scale unmatched by any other HIV NGO. The real TAC is [over 200 branches] varying in size from a couple of dozen up to 200 members, who are working in their communities, trying to do condom workshops, educate healthcare workers, gather information on the extent and availability of health services, build relations with doctors, nurses and administrators, help people access services, and educate communities.

This mobilisation at grassroots level has helped the TAC to keep pace with the realities of inequality and violence that are driving the HIV/AIDS epidemic and its devastating impacts on communities across South Africa.

Gender, power, violence and HIV/AIDS

Across the southern African region, existing gender-related norms condone men's violence against women, grant men the power to initiate and dictate the terms of sex, and make it extremely difficult for women to protect themselves from either HIV or violence.[2] As a result, the HIV/AIDS epidemic has a markedly disproportionate impact on women's lives. A recent study revealed that young women are much more likely to be infected than their male peers, with women making up 77 per cent of the 10 per cent of South African youth between the ages of 15 and 24 who are infected with HIV/AIDS (Pettifor, Rees and Steffenson 2004).

Women's greater vulnerability to HIV/AIDS is explained to a great degree by the high levels of sexual and domestic violence perpetuated against them. South Africa has the highest per capita rate of reported rape in the world (Dunkle et al. 2004). As elsewhere, women are most at risk of sexual and physical violence from men that they know. Research conducted by the Medical Research Council in 2004 shows that a woman is killed by her intimate partner in South Africa every six days (Mathews et al. 2004; see also Chapter 2 in this volume). A study of more than 1 500 South African women published in *The Lancet* in May 2004 shows that women in abusive relationships have a higher risk of HIV infection. The study reports that women who are beaten or dominated by their partners are nearly 50 per cent more likely to become infected with HIV than women in non-violent households (Dunkle et al. 2004). A review of research articles from 1996 to 2002 found nine studies showing that women who experienced sexual coercion were more at risk of HIV transmission (Manfrin-Ledet and Porche 2003).

In South Africa, the fact that women are often economically dependent on men exacerbates their vulnerability to violence and to HIV/AIDS and its associated impacts, making it difficult for women to leave abusive and/or sexually coercive relationships. In his book *Inequality in South Africa*, Stephen Gelb examines the precarious economic situation of many South African women (2003). He notes that women's participation in the labour force is much lower than men's. In 1995, only 17 per cent of African females were in wage employment, compared with 43 per cent of African men, and only 45 per cent of white women were in the labour force, compared with 63 per cent of white men. Despite the changes in government and the significant increase in the number of women represented at government level, Gelb argues that the gender gap in real wages has widened substantially. He observes that in 1999, for example, women's hourly wage as a percentage of men's dropped from 77.9 per cent to 65.6 per cent.

Women are also confronted with many obstacles in bringing the perpetrators of violence against them to justice. Many women have little faith in a criminal justice system that produces one of the lowest conviction rates for domestic and sexual violence in the world. The failures of the criminal justice system to adequately respond to violence against women reflect society's collusion with such violence and permit male violence to continue with impunity.

Despite alarmingly high levels of rape and HIV/AIDS, post-exposure prophylaxis (PEP) is unavailable to many rape survivors. The South African non-governmental organisation (NGO) GenderLinks found PEP readily available at only 43 per cent of the institutions it visited in 2003: 84 per cent of hospitals, but only 15 per cent of clinics. This has serious implications, given that many women have limited access to hospitals and PEP must be administered within 72 hours of exposure in order to be effective. Studies also indicate that only 30 per cent of staff caring for rape survivors had received specialised training on dealing with rape (Christofides et al. 2005).

However, while commentators agree that state and communal responses to violence against women remain deeply problematic, violence against particular groups of men and its role in heightening their vulnerability are almost entirely neglected in the public discourse on violence, gender and HIV/AIDS. Homophobic violence against gay men and other men who have sex with men is ignored or condoned and this drives these men away from needed services. Male survivors of violence can expect little help from the criminal justice system – indeed, they face the risk of being further violated by the system itself, not only from the widespread homophobia among the staff of its institutions, but also from the possibility of direct violence from police and other law enforcement officers. Prisoners' vulnerability to rape and sexual assault, and the impact of such violence on their vulnerability to HIV infection, are also only now beginning to receive the attention they deserve (see Chapter 8 for more on prisons and HIV/AIDS).

Civil society responses to gender-based violence and HIV/AIDS
Despite the high levels of gender-based violence experienced by both men and women in South Africa, there has been a widespread failure on the part of civil society to

effectively address the gendered dimensions of HIV/AIDS in South Africa. Women's advocacy organisations have had limited impact in improving the state's response to violence against women or addressing gender inequalities. In an article published in the *Mail & Guardian*, Marlise Richter argues:

> The AIDS crisis necessitates a blazing, outspoken feminist response that includes challenging the slow implementation of anti-retrovirals, the preposterous levels of gender-based violence, the deficient care of rape survivors, the far-reaching implications of the prevention of mother-to-child transmission programme and the hopelessly inadequate prevention responses to the ways in which young women and girls contract HIV. (Richter 2005a)

However, with the exception of the demonstrations in front of the Johannesburg High Court during the Jacob Zuma rape trial, there is little evidence of this feminist response. Rather than the sort of militancy suggested by Richter and others, Shireen Hassin argues that the post-1994 women's movement has opted for inclusion in the democratic state, producing an elite-oriented leadership within the movement that has rarely used collective action as the basis to build a strong mass movement of women (2004).

The South African government's response to gender-based violence has also been ineffectual and is an example of progressive legislation undermined by poor enforcement. The National Crime Prevention Strategy of 1996 established violence against women as a national priority and in 1998 activists within the government and civil society were able to ensure passage through parliament of a progressive and far-reaching Domestic Violence Act (DVA) intended 'to convey that the State is committed to the elimination of domestic violence' (preamble to *Domestic Violence Act 116 of 1998*). Unfortunately, expressions of commitment by the government have not been matched by the financial and human resources needed to implement change.

Two oversight and co-ordinating bodies, the Commission on Gender Equality (CGE) and the Human Rights Commission (HRC), have been established by the government since 1994 to advance gender equality and human rights. But they have offered only muted and infrequent criticism of the government's ineffectual efforts to prevent violence against women, or to address the gendered dimensions of HIV/AIDS. The TAC has criticised this lack of engagement. In a memorandum handed to the CGE in April 2003, the TAC rebuked the CGE, saying:

> We would have expected the CGE to lead the struggle for the prevention and treatment of HIV/AIDS. Instead, you have been silent on the reproductive rights of women who desire to minimise HIV transmission . . . you ignore the public calls that government should operationalise a plan to ensure that women and children have access to antiretroviral post exposure prophylaxis. You stand by silently while women die. (Richter 2005b)

Growing commitment: The TAC, gender and HIV/AIDS

Over the years, the TAC itself has been criticised for its apparent lack of focus on the gendered dimensions of HIV/AIDS. This was compounded by the perception that the TAC's leadership was predominantly male. Its successful PMTCT campaign was criticised in some quarters for focusing only on preventing vertical transmission from mothers to their infant children, rather than demanding access to treatment for women. Similarly, the TAC received criticism for not advocating for PEP, without comparable demands for a comprehensive package of care for rape survivors. Legal scholars have also asked important questions about whether the organisation did not miss a critical opportunity to advance a feminist jurisprudence when the TAC framed the PMTCT case in terms of a right to healthcare, rather than in terms of women's rights to sexual and reproductive health (Richter 2006).

While these criticisms are partly valid, a closer analysis of the organisation reveals a commitment to addressing the gender inequalities underlying the HIV/AIDS epidemic. Nearly 70 per cent of the TAC's members are women and most elected and appointed positions in the national office are filled by women. The organisation's 2005 National Congress was themed 'Women and People with HIV Leadership for a People's Health Service' and saw the organisation's rank-and-file membership elect women into 50 per cent of senior leadership positions. The congress recognised that the TAC needed to provide leadership positions for women and PLWHA.

The TAC's grassroots response to the rape and murder of Lorna Mlofana in Khayelitsha in 2003 also illustrates a commitment to addressing gender-based violence at the community level. On 13 December 2003, 22-year-old TAC member, Lorna Mlofana, was raped by a group of five men outside a shebeen in the Town

Two area of Khayelitsha, a sprawling formal and informal settlement of 500 000 people, just outside Cape Town. When she disclosed that she was HIV-positive, they murdered her. The TAC made a firm commitment to ensure that the people responsible would be held accountable in the criminal justice system. Phumeza, a friend of Lorna's and a fellow TAC activist, describes her response to Lorna's death: 'Because Lorna was part of us, we felt we had to take action. We had to ensure that there's justice for people like us – poor people living with HIV and AIDS.'[3] Mandla Majola, the TAC co-ordinator for Khayelitsha, remembers his response: 'She was an ordinary person in Khayelitsha wanting to make a difference. One had to respond.' Based on prior experiences, however, Mandla knew that the 'TAC would have to push and stretch the justice system. If we had not put pressure on the police, nothing would have been done.'

Spearheaded by Lorna's friends, the TAC began to run workshops throughout Town Two, an area that had previously been a no-go area for the TAC because of its high levels of violent crime. One female TAC activist, then sixteen years old, describes the impact of this outreach: 'Initially people were afraid to support us, but then they gradually found the courage to become involved and we held a mini-march through Town Two.' In a place where people are used to murderers being released, she says that the community saw that this case was different: 'People saw how serious it was through our activism.'

The TAC activists quickly became targets for intimidation by the perpetrators and their friends. One of them came home one evening to find that friends of the perpetrators had come looking for her. One member of the Khayelitsha branch remembers that 'they would say "we will see you in the community"'. The TAC informed the police of the threats and stepped up its community education and mobilisation activities in Town Two. Together with a growing number of community members, the TAC continued to pressure the police to take action and used its connections in the community to secure the evidence necessary to arrest the men involved. The TAC then mobilised large demonstrations at the court hearings, opposed bail and reminded the judge that as a public servant, he was accountable to the community.

On the anniversary of Lorna's death, with the perpetrators awaiting trial, the TAC organised a rally in Khayelitsha to remember Lorna and to continue to educate the community about the importance of taking action to address violence against women. At the rally, the TAC presented a petition to the Department of Health

(DoH), drawing attention to the fact that rape survivors in Khayelitsha had to travel long distances to reach critical emergency services and calling for the immediate establishment of a full-service rape crisis centre in Khayelitsha. In response, the Simelela Rape Crisis Centre was established in Site B and now provides previously unavailable counselling and PEP to rape survivors. In the first six months it was open, 442 rape survivors sought treatment from the Simelela Centre. This is more than the total number of rapes reported in Khayelitsha for the whole of 2003–04 (Thom 2006).

After numerous postponements by the Magistrates' Court in Khayelitsha, finally, on 8 December 2005, the Court found the first accused guilty of murder and rape, and the second accused guilty of attempted murder. On 16 February 2006, the Cape High Court sentenced the first accused to life in prison for murder and a concurrent ten-year sentence for rape. The second accused was sentenced to ten years in prison for assault.

The impact of Lorna's case

> In Khayelitsha people are coming forward now to report rape cases, and I think that is because of our community mobilisation efforts to show that rape is wrong. People are also now getting assistance from Simelela, which is open 24 hours. If you go to Simelela and access [the] counselling service, there is a police officer who is based in this centre; then you don't have to go to the police station to report the case. The police officer will take your statement and open a case. So we are promoting Simelela throughout our communities here in Khayelitsha. (Mandla Majola, TAC co-ordinator for Khayelitsha)

The impact of the TAC's activism related to Lorna's case has been significant. Pointing to the limitations inherent in responding to rape only after it has occurred, Mandla emphasises the need to work in the community to prevent rape. With a view to such violence prevention, the TAC locally has worked with the police to address the problem of illegal shebeens. There are about 55 legally operating shebeens in Khayelitsha, but some 500 illegal pubs. With the understanding that heavy drinking is often a prelude to, if not a direct cause of, sexual violence, the TAC is working with the police to reduce the number of drinking venues in the area. Mandla Majola adds that:

We have also formed a partnership with Simelela and Masibambane, a drama group doing a play on rape, on what we should do to prevent rape and to get services after you have been raped. We have targeted ten primary schools in Khayelitsha where they go and do the play, and we want to ensure that each primary school gets to see the play. Kids can begin to understand what rape is, what they can do to prevent it, and if it has happened, why they must go forward to get services that are being provided.

The case also had a major impact on the TAC and its membership. Outrage about Lorna's murder and the criminal justice system's reluctant response galvanised TAC members in Khayelitsha and across the country to deepen their understanding of both gender-based violence and the inadequacies of the criminal justice system's approach to addressing it. The case opened up discussions among women within the organisation about gender-based violence and gradually created awareness that many female activists are also survivors of domestic and sexual violence. Women involved described the ways in which their activism informed their growing critical consciousness, saying, for example, 'We didn't know there were things happening to us that were also rape. Being involved in educating the community gave us a clear understanding.' Another Khayelitsha-based TAC activist says, 'It also opened my eyes. I used to blame rape victims.' As discussed in the next section, the case has also prompted men within the TAC to begin to address their responsibility for stopping the violence.

The activism surrounding the case also shifted the organisation away from an ideological commitment to addressing violence against women to a much more deeply felt commitment and as a personal issue affecting many TAC staff and members – both as a human rights issue and as a major cause of the spread and impact of HIV/AIDS. During Jacob Zuma's rape trial in 2006, for example, male and female activists picketed the streets outside the court to demand that the woman involved be given a fair hearing. The TAC also issued press statements condemning the intimidation tactics used by Zuma's supporters, arguing that violence against women constitutes a daily attack on the dignity and equality of women, as well as on South Africa's social values.

The TAC has also carried out a series of internal meetings on gender and on women's rights and led a number of marches that have emphasised the relationship between violence against women and HIV prevention, including those at the 2005 International Microbicides Conference in Cape Town and the rally held in the Western Cape on 16 June 2005. Gender inequalities and gender-based violence were also a significant focus of the TAC's participation at both the second UN General Assembly Special Session on AIDS (UNGASS) and at the Toronto International AIDS Conference. At UNGASS, the TAC's representatives – all women, the majority of whom were HIV-positive – spoke to the General Assembly about the centrality of addressing violence against women in all HIV/AIDS prevention work.

Men, gender, HIV/AIDS and the TAC

Lorna's case prompted the TAC to incorporate a strong focus on supporting men to oppose gender-based violence and to take public stands for gender equality. As part of its commitment to addressing gender inequalities, the TAC has supported a number of Khayelitsha-based activists in forming two structures for men and women that encourage reflection and ultimately action: Positive Women United and Positive Men United (POMU). Mandla Majola described his motivation for supporting the development of a TAC structure for men:

> Men must be involved in the campaign against violence. We must condemn the violence that men do. We have to go to men's forums, football clubs and sheebens to educate each other. We also have to go to big football matches like Kaizer Chiefs and Sundowns because they are dominated by men. We should also involve the youth. For example, during the circumcision period young men should be taught why abuse of women is wrong. Men struggle to find their dignity in Khayelitsha. We have high unemployment. So many men feel useless. They use alcohol and drugs to try to cure their frustrations. Then they vent their anger on women because they think women won't fight back. We need to give men their dignity back. (Kamkam and Geffen 2006)

POMU has now spread into many of the TAC's branches across the Western Cape. One POMU member, a treatment literacy activist acknowledges that he was previously abusive and was arrested for stabbing his girlfriend. He believes that his activism has been transformative. As he says, 'What happened to Lorna changed my behaviour. It educated me about the need to negotiate and discuss sex. When my girlfriend says no, I have to listen.'

Other TAC-related initiatives have sought to encourage more caring and responsible forms of masculinity. In Gauteng, the Western Cape and the Eastern Cape, the TAC has worked together with the Men as Partners (MAP) network to mobilise men for gender justice and men within the TAC have participated in a number of MAP network workshops, marches and community education events (Peacock and Levack 2004). Reflecting this, men within TAC who are active within the organisation's MAP programme are attempting to integrate MAP representatives into local government structures, such as the Ekhuruleni AIDS Stakeholders Forum and the Ekhuruleni AIDS Council on Johannesburg's East Rand. In this way, they hope to use these structures to ensure that gender equality work with men gets mainstreamed into all HIV/AIDS work in the area.

There is also a growing commitment within the TAC to recognise and address men's health needs. Research shows that it is often men who are disadvantaged by gender norms when it comes to accessing services. Khululeka, an all-men's support group formed in Gugulethu by men involved with the TAC, for example, was formed by men who saw that men were not participating in support groups and arrived at clinics only when they were seriously ill (Robins 2006). In Ekhuruleni, the TAC participates in a monthly HIV/AIDS stakeholders' forum and in each of Ekhuruleni's Customer Care Centres to monitor service delivery. In an interview conducted by the authors with TAC Ekhuruleni activists in May 2006, they told us that in order to ensure that these structures work to engage men and to increase men's utilisation of HIV/AIDS services, TAC activists are working hard to make sure that each community structure has a MAP representative.

The TAC's approach recognises the gendering of both women and men, and not only seeks to hold men accountable for the ways in which they sustain gender inequalities through their attitudes and behaviour, but also to address the ways in which they are harmed by gender norms. This dual emphasis on both challenging men and supporting them in change is often difficult to balance. The need to hold men accountable for their sexist attitudes and behaviour has sometimes been seen as compromising the effort to reach out to men and engage them by talking about their needs, yet both approaches are clearly necessary. As the TAC deepens its gender-based work with men, through POMU and other structures, it will face the continued challenge of translating its dual emphasis into practice.

The strengths of the TAC model

A key element of the TAC's success is that, unlike most organisations in South Africa, the TAC is able to infuse gender activism with the vision, strategic skills and collective power necessary to improve the state's currently inadequate response to the gendered dimensions of HIV/AIDS. The TAC's response to the rape and murder of Lorna Mlofana and its recent focus on AIDS prevention at UNGASS also demonstrate the organisation's ability to mobilise thousands of people to make insistent demands that state and civil society organisations challenge the gender roles, relations and inequalities that exacerbate the spread and impact of HIV/AIDS. This combination of grassroots mobilisation and national-level protest with international visibility has given the TAC significant influence in shaping policy discourse and leverage in developing policy, whether on issues of HIV prevention, AIDS treatment, or gender-based violence. A further lesson from the TAC's experience is the importance of combining dissent with a willingness to work strategically with the government at all levels, where there is an opportunity to both push a policy agenda from the inside and ensure its implementation.

Such a twin-track approach, used so successfully in relation to national AIDS treatment roll-out, has significant potential for the TAC and other organisations in their work on gender-based violence. This is already beginning to happen. In Khayelitsha, TAC activists have marched on many occasions to demand that the police take action in cases of reported domestic violence. Following the AIDS Law Project (ALP) and TAC's successful lawsuit against the Department of Correctional Services (DCS) demanding access to treatment for prisoners, the TAC engaged in civil disobedience and occupied the Cape Town offices of the HRC to force the DCS to comply with the court ruling. To date, gender equality activists have not engaged in this kind of civil disobedience.

Other TAC strategies provide important lessons for gender activists. For instance, there are important lessons to be learned from the work of the Joint Civil Society Monitoring Forum (JCSMF). The JCSMF was established by the TAC and the ALP to monitor treatment roll-out. The JCSMF consists of service providers, NGOs involved in treatment delivery and advocacy and a range of legal advocacy and research organisations, who together track and report on the roll-out to keep the pressure on the government to deliver on its commitments. Faced with poor implementation of the DVA, evidence of ongoing disregard and sometimes violence at the hands of police, a model such as the JCSMF allows activists to track progress from arrest to prosecution and conviction, and to hold the criminal justice system accountable in some of the same ways that the JCSMF does with the DoH. Similarly, this model could be used to track access to PEP among victims of gender-based violence.

At the same time, the TAC's experience of partnering with local government structures, such as district AIDS councils, community policing forums, clinic committees and youth structures can also be applied to work on ensuring service delivery at the local level. This includes legal, health and welfare services for the survivors of violence, as well as HIV/AIDS service delivery for men. The TAC's success in the Lorna Mlofana case, for instance, has led to closer working relationships with organisations working against gender-based violence. Together with staff from Rape Crisis, the South African Police Services (SAPS) and the Departments of Health and Social Services, the TAC now co-ordinates a monthly meeting to support the new Simelela Sexual Assault Centre in Khayelitsha.

Future directions within the TAC

The TAC is confronted with the challenge of implementing its commitment to internal reform. While its effort to bring women into leadership positions has provided a model for other social justice movements, the TAC has also experienced internal tensions related to its efforts to promote gender equality within the organisation. Some men in the organisation have, at times, resisted change and undermined efforts to build women's leadership. With a national leadership comprised mostly of women, but with mid-level management at the provincial and district level made up mostly of men, national directives perceived by some men as threatening have sometimes been blocked or undermined (telephone interviews with Gordon Mthembu, Ekhuruleni district co-ordinator and Phologolo Ramothwala, Limpopo provincial co-ordinator, 27 April 2006). Working through such reactions and expanding the constituency for gender equality that does exist within the organisation will require not simply policy directives, but also structured opportunities for men and women to discuss gender equality at a personal, as well as a political level. Participation in the MAP network is a significant step in the right direction in terms of doing the gender work that is necessary to realise the TAC's feminist commitments.

At the same time, the TAC's work with men also has the potential to inspire existing men's initiatives to focus more on direct action and activism than has been the case to date among organisations that have had an almost exclusive focus on running workshops aimed at behaviour change – without paying much attention to what happens afterwards (for an overview of emerging work with men in South Africa, see Peacock and Botha 2006). The example set by the TAC in Khayelitsha may encourage groups like MAP to emphasise more strategic approaches, such as advocacy aimed at winning concrete services for survivors of violence, as happened with the Simelela Sexual Assault Centre, or demanding that the criminal justice system hold perpetrators accountable. To achieve this, the TAC will need to make its work with men more visible and commit to train and mentor other organisations attempting to work with men to promote gender equality.

Ultimately, the challenge for the TAC's gender activism, as for other social justice movements addressing inequalities and gender-based violence, remains to build a movement that can begin to transform the beliefs, practices and institutions that obstruct gender justice. Richter frames the critical question that remains unanswered:

> It is arguable that many HIV/AIDS programmes in South Africa focus on the amelioration of women's worsening position in society because of the epidemic – for example the calls for safer sex and other prevention programmes, the development of an AIDS vaccine and microbicides, the provision of home-based care, and the provision of ARVs – be it in the form of prevention or treatment. These programmes aspire and in some ways fulfil women's practical gender interests. The question is whether they can do more. Can these same programmes also serve as an effective vehicle for providing for women's strategic gender interests? Can they be used to fundamentally question women's position in society, patriarchal notions of sex and the gender roles assumed by the different sexes? This is the challenge the epidemic poses to us, and the opportunity it offers. (2006)

Conclusion
While the TAC is best known for its much publicised PMTCT campaign and its efforts to secure access to ARVs for all HIV-positive South Africans, it is increasingly trying to not only address the gendered dimensions of HIV/AIDS and to secure PEP for rape survivors, but also to demand justice for survivors of sexual violence. It has been able to draw on its unique combination of grassroots mobilisation and visibility, as well as its large national membership, to raise awareness about the gender underpinnings of the epidemic and to address the dynamics driving both men's

and women's vulnerability to HIV and AIDS. These attributes have given the TAC significant influence in shaping policy discourse and have placed it in a strategically strong position to address the on-the-ground realities of ordinary South Africans.

The TAC's success in forwarding both the treatment and gender agendas illustrates the important oversight and implementing role that civil society can play in addressing the spread and effects of the epidemic and also provides important lessons for other civil society actors. It also underscores the potential value of civil society-government partnerships, which provide opportunities for civil society to engage with the government on policy and implementation, while also allowing under-resourced government departments to tap into the commitment and organisational resources available to movements such as the TAC.

On a more personal note, the TAC's recent efforts provide hope that social change is possible. This has been especially true for me, Thoko Budaza. My own history of sexual abuse as a child and rape as an adult, and the utter failure of the criminal justice system to deal with my many experiences of violence, is the story of so many South African women. Yet I am one of the lucky few who had access to PEP, minimising the risk of my contracting HIV from the rapist. The work by TAC activists to secure justice for their colleague and comrade Lorna Mlofana following her rape and murder, and the knowledge that the TAC had helped to secure PEP for rape survivors, served as a source of much-needed inspiration for me during the weeks of nausea, debilitating depression and police inaction in the weeks following the rape. Indeed, the TAC's readiness and capacity to mobilise its membership in the struggle for gender justice gives us all hope that patriarchal notions of sex and women's subordination can be ended and that gender relations between women and men can be truly transformed.

Notes

1. The TAC is currently conducting an audit of its membership to determine the exact number of active members.
2. Rachel Jewkes's extensive writings on gender-based violence and HIV include the following useful pieces: Jewkes et al. 2001, Jewkes 2002 and Jewkes, Levin and Penn-Kekana 2003.
3. All quotes in this case study are drawn from three focus group discussions held in the TAC Khayelitsha district office in March, April and May of 2006.

References

Annas, George. 2003. 'The Right to Health and the Nevirapine Case in South Africa'. *New England Journal of Medicine* 348(8): 750–54.

Christofides, Nicola J., Rachel K. Jewkes, Naomi Webster, Loveday Penn-Kekana, Naeema Abrahams and Lorna J. Martin. 2005. '"Other Patients Are Really in Need of Medical Attention": The Quality of Health Services for Rape Survivors in South Africa'. *Bulletin of the World Health Organization* 83: 495–502.

Department of Health (DoH). 2003. 'Operational Plan for Comprehensive HIV and AIDS Care, Management and Treatment for South Africa'. Pretoria: DoH.

De Waal, Alex. 2006. *AIDS and Power: Why There Is No Political Crisis – Yet*. London and New York: Zed Books.

Dunkle, Kristin, Rachel Jewkes, Heather Brown, Glenda Gray, James McIntrye and Sioban Harlow. 2004. 'Gender-Based Violence, Relationship Power, and Risk of HIV Infection in Women Attending Antenatal Clinics in South Africa'. *The Lancet* 363(9 419): 1 415–421.

Friedman, Steven and Shauna Mottiar. 2005. 'A Rewarding Engagement? The Treatment Action Campaign and the Politics of HIV/AIDS'. *Politics and Society* 33(4): 511–65.

Gelb, Stephan. 2003. *Inequality in South Africa: Nature, Causes and Responses*. Johannesburg: The Edge Institute.

GenderLinks. 2003. 'Report on the PEP Talk Campaign Conducted during the Sixteen Days of Activism on Gender Violence'. Available at http://www.genderlinks.org.za/item.php?i_id=126, accessed 21 December 2007.

Hassin, Shireen. 2004. 'Voices, Hierarchies and Spaces: Reconfiguring the Women's Movement in Democratic South Africa'. Research report, Centre for Civil Society and School of Development Studies, University of KwaZulu-Natal.

Jewkes, Rachel. 2002. 'Intimate Partner Violence: Causes and Prevention'. *The Lancet* 359(9 315): 1 423–429.

Jewkes, Rachel, Jonathan Levin and Loveday Penn-Kekana. 2003. 'Gender Inequalities, Intimate Partner Violence and HIV Preventive Practices: Findings of a South African Cross-Sectional Study'. *Social Science and Medicine* 56(1): 125–34.

Jewkes, Rachel, Caesar Vundule, Fidelia Majorah and Esmé Jordaan. 2001. 'Relationship Dynamics and Teenage Pregnancy in South Africa'. *Social Science and Medicine* 52(5): 733–44.

Kamkam, Vathiswa and Nathan Geffen. 2006. '"Restoring Men's Dignity": An Interview with Mandla Majola'. *Equal Treatment*, June 2006. Available at http://www.tac.org.za/documents/et20.pdf, accessed 21 December 2007.

Khan, Farook. 2005. 'Prison Inmates Starve to Get ARVs'. *Independent Online* 19 July. Available at http://www.iol.co.za/general/newsview.php?art_id=vn20050719084433438C384164&click_id=2624&set_id=1, accessed 16 June 2006.

Manfrin-Ledet, Linda and Demetrius Porche. 2003. 'The State of Science: Violence and HIV Infection in Women'. *Journal of the Association of Nurses in AIDS Care* 14(6): 56–68.

Mathews, Shanaaz, Naeemah Abrahams, Lorna Martin, Lisa Vetten, Lize van der Merwe and Rachel Jewkes. 2004. *Every Six Hours a Woman is Killed by her Intimate Partner: A National Study of Female Homicide in South Africa*. Tygerberg: Gender and Health Research Group and Medical Research Council.

Mbali, Mandisa. 2005. 'The Treatment Action Campaign and the History of Rights-Based, Patient-Driven HIV/AIDS Activism in South Africa'. Research Report 29, University of KwaZulu-Natal, Centre for Civil Society.

Mosoetsa, Sarah. 2005. 'Compromised Communities and Re-emerging Civic Engagement in Mpumalanga Township, Durban, KwaZulu-Natal'. *Journal of Southern African Studies* 31(4): 857–73.

Peacock, Dean and Mbuyisela Botha. 2006. 'The New Gender Platforms and Fatherhood'. In *Baba: Men and Fatherhood in South Africa*, ed. Linda Richter and Robert Morrell. Cape Town: Human Sciences Research Council Press.

Peacock, Dean and Andrew Levack. 2004. 'The Men as Partners Program in South Africa: Reaching Men to End Gender-Based Violence and Promote Sexual and Reproductive Health'. *International Journal of Men's Health* 3(3): 173–88.

Pettifor, Audrey, Helen Rees and Annie Steffenson. 2004. *HIV and Sexual Behaviour among Young South Africans: A National Survey of 15–24 Year Olds*. Johannesburg: University of the Witwatersrand Press.

Richter, Marlise. 2005a. 'A New Feminism'. *Mail & Guardian* 9 December.

———. 2005b. 'Socio-Economic Citizenship, Women and HIV/AIDS in South Africa'. Unpublished paper.

———. 2006. 'How Do the Blind Spots in AIDS Discourse Affect the Experiences of Not Only HIV-Positive Women, But Women in General?' Paper presented at the TAC women's reference group meeting, Gordon's Bay, 17–18 March.

Robins, Steven. 2004. 'Long Live Zackie, Long Live: AIDS Activism, Science and Citizenship after Apartheid'. *Journal of Southern African Studies* 30(3): 651–72.

———. 2006. 'Khululeka – From Social Movement to Men's Support Group: A Case Study of AIDS Activism in Gugulethu, Cape Town'. *New Agenda: South African Journal of Social and Economic Policy* 21: 29–33.

Thom, Anso. 2006. 'Disturbing Picture of Sexual Violence in Khayelitsha'. *Health-e News* 31 March.

Treatment Action Campaign (TAC). 2005. 'Political Report 2003/05 for the Third National Congress'. Available at http://www.tac.org.za/documents/NationalCongressDocumentation2005.doc, accessed 21 December 2007.

———. 2006. 'Massive Youth March for HIV Prevention'. 15 June. Available at http://www.tac.org.za/nl20060615.html, accessed 18 June 2006.

5

The Public Education Sector and HIV/AIDS[1]

————•————

Karl Peltzer

Introduction

There has been growing attention to the issue of HIV/AIDS and its potential impact on education. A number of research projects have provided a very gloomy picture. A report of the United Nations (International) Children's (Emergency) Fund (UNICEF) in 1999 highlighted that the epidemic would have a particular impact on the education sector. In 2000, a report by the United Nations Educational, Scientific and Cultural Organisation (UNESCO), addressed the growing anxiety that in the most heavily affected countries, HIV-infection rates were highest among teachers (Kelly 2000).

In South Africa, conjecture has led to conclusions that educators are dying in large numbers as a result of HIV/AIDS, prompting concerns that the epidemic contributes significantly to attrition of public educators. Indeed, the education sector is in a precarious situation as a result of the HIV/AIDS epidemic, if not simply because the quality of today's educational institutions will affect the future. Thus, 'as governments contend with increasing demands on social and economic services while coping with weakened capacity due to slow growth, it is likely that the "developmental state" in South Africa may not be realised. The result could be increased vulnerability among poor, who are dependent on the state's capacity to deliver health, water, housing, and education services.' (CCR 2006, 6)

The relationship between AIDS and the education sector is circular – as the epidemic worsens, the education sector is damaged, which in turn is likely to increase the incidence of HIV transmission. There are numerous ways in which AIDS can affect education, but equally there are many ways in which education can contribute to controlling AIDS. The extent to which schools and other educational institutions are able to continue functioning will influence how well and how quickly societies will eventually recover from the HIV/AIDS epidemic.

It was for these reasons that in 2004 and 2005, the Education Labour Relations Council (ELRC), a body comprising the South African Department of Education and educators' unions, including the South African Democratic Teachers' Union (SADTU), National Professional Teachers' Organisation of South Africa (NAPTOSA), Suid-Afrikaanse Onderwyserunie (SAOU) and the National Teachers' Union (NATU), commissioned the Human Sciences Research Council (HSRC) to undertake a study to establish the facts about the impact of HIV/AIDS on the education sector. The aim of the study was to determine: (a) the extent of HIV among educators in public schools and student educators; (b) the factors driving the HIV epidemic among educators and student educators; and (c) make recommendations for interventions to mitigate the impact of HIV/AIDS on this population.

Much has been written about the importance of education to building literacy and providing life skills as a strategy for strengthening the effectiveness of HIV prevention. Since HIV/AIDS mainly affects productive adults, education has also been cited as an important sector for addressing human resource shortfalls. Based on the ELRC/HSRC study, this chapter sets out to share empirical evidence on self-reported measures of HIV status within South Africa's public education system. It aims to answer two basic, but important questions. First, what is the prevalence of HIV/AIDS among educators in public schools, training colleges and students in educator training? Second, what are the factors driving the HIV/AIDS epidemic among educators?

The need for evidence

According to Paul Bennel, there were about 2.75 million teachers in primary and secondary schools in the 49 countries of sub-Saharan Africa in the late 1990s (2003). These educators accounted for more than one-third of public servants in all the countries of the region. Comprising such a significant percentage of the public sector means that educators are, in many ways, the bedrock of development in these countries. This makes it important to ascertain what the HIV/AIDS prevalence is in these populations and how the epidemic impacts on educators, who are in turn, responsible for preparing tomorrow's engineers, scientists, doctors, nurses, economists, mathematicians, etc. Despite the importance of this sector, not a single national study on HIV prevalence among educators had been undertaken to establish the extent of the problem and its determinants until the ELRC/HSRC survey in

2004–05. Most of the studies that had been published previously were based on projections and conjecture.

Some earlier studies were premised on a theory that proposes that HIV/AIDS affects the supply of and the demand for education. The supply is affected through the reduction in the number of skilled educators, administrators and other education personnel (Badcock-Walters and Görgens 2001). AIDS-related illness and deaths of teachers deprive learners of the sector's most experienced senior teachers and managers, including Science and Mathematics teachers (Coombe 2002). Prior to their deaths, many educators are likely to be absent from teaching – hence their colleagues have to take on their responsibilities, especially in poorly resourced schools that do not have substitute teachers. A lack of HIV-related workplace polices compounds the problem, as there often is no sick pay, no access to HIV/AIDS treatment and inadequate teacher replacement policies (Coombe 2002). Once ill educators die, their colleagues spend time going to funerals, thus increasing absenteeism from school. This leads to increased workload and poor working conditions for educators in the most heavily affected schools (SADTU 2003). Furthermore, there are costly implications for the maintenance of good quality education and the overall impact on education systems. The demand for education is affected by a reduction in supply within the context of HIV/AIDS.

While there may be reduction in the quality of education, the pandemic could also reduce the pool of skilled and semi-skilled workers in other sectors, such as agriculture, finance, entrepreneurial business, transportation, construction, the arts, law and medicine. Presumably, it will become even more critical to have an education system in place that meets the needs of developing societies in these sectors. At the same time, increasing numbers of orphans (see Chapter 7 in this volume) and the impact on households in rural areas (see Chapter 6) is likely to increase the need and urgency for a strong and sustainable education system. Because of the critical role that educators play in the education system and in society, it is imperative that empirical evidence on the epidemiology of HIV/AIDS among teachers be generated. Such information is crucial in planning human resources for the education system, and in developing appropriate HIV prevention and care strategies.

A note on methodology

The ELRC/HSRC study was a cross-sectional survey in South Africa among a nationally representative sample of 20 626 educators and a sample of 1 056 student educators. The survey employed the second-generation surveillance method that combines the measurement of behavioural and biological indicators (Shisana et al. 2005, xv).

Findings of the ELRC/HRSC study: Educators
Demographic and socio-economic characteristics

The demographic and socio-economic profiles of educators in the sample indicate that educators are largely female (68 per cent). The majority of educators are married (61 per cent). Over three-quarters of the sample were black people (77 per cent), while less than 5 per cent of the sample were Asians, which is a reflection of the demographic characteristics of South Africa. The observed age profile of educators in the sample suggests that nearly half of the sample were in the 35–44 age group, while less than 2 per cent were between 18 and 24 years old. A negligible proportion was in the age group of 55 years old or older (5 per cent).

Self-reported socio-economic status and income distribution suggest that these educators were well off financially and generally well qualified, with long years of teaching experience. About half of the educators in the sample had a first degree at tertiary level or a higher qualification. Approximately 70 per cent had at least ten years of teaching experience. About 94 per cent of educators reported that the Department of Education employed them, while the remaining 6 per cent are in governing-body appointments.

Only 27 per cent of educators in the sample reported having housing subsidies and 67.8 per cent of the educators reported that they were members of a medical aid fund. The majority of educators surveyed are members of a trade union (89 per cent). The findings show that there are proportionately more female and male black educators in the low-income category, compared with educators in other race groups. On the other hand, there are proportionately fewer male white educators in the medium-income category than male educators in other race groups.

HIV prevalence

Blood specimens for HIV testing were obtained from 17 088 educators. The results show that 12.7 per cent of educators were HIV-positive. This percentage includes educators in all provinces in South Africa and people of both sexes and all age and racial groups. It is estimated that the 12.7 per cent HIV prevalence is equivalent to 45 307 educators nationally. The true figure lies somewhere between 42 809 on the low end and 47 804 at the higher end. These results confirm what Peter Badcock-

Walters and Marelize Görgens reported in 2001: HIV/AIDS affects the supply of education by reducing the number of skilled educators.

Women are generally more vulnerable to HIV infection because of biological factors, as well as their lower socio-economic status (see Chapter 2 in this volume). It is thus no surprise that in the general population of South Africa, women have higher HIV prevalence ratios than men. In this study, however, the male and female educators had almost similar HIV prevalence, 12.7 per cent and 12.8 per cent respectively, as can be seen in Table 5.1. Furthermore, the results show that HIV

Table 5.1 HIV prevalence by various demographic characteristics of public sector educators in ELRC/HSRC study, South Africa, 2004.

Characteristics	Number surveyed	HIV-positive (percentage)	95 per cent confidence interval (CI)
Total	**17 088**	**12.7**	**12.0–13.5**
Sex			
Men	5 455	12.7	11.6–13.9
Women	11 621	12.8	12.0–13.6
Race			
Black	12 022	16.3	15.5–17.1
White	2 165	0.4	0.2–0.8
Coloured	2 309	0.7	0.4–1.3
Indian	533	1.0	0.5–2.1
Age			
< 24	240	6.5	3.4–12.0
25–34	4 282	21.4	19.9–23.0
35–44	7 443	12.8	11.8–13.8
45–54	4 274	5.8	5.0–6.7
55 and above	842	3.1	2.1–4.6
Marital status			
Married, civil	3 329	7.9	6.9–9.1
Married, traditional (*ilobola*/dowry)	635	15.4	12.5–18.9
Married, religious	3 288	5.5	4.5–6.7
Married, civil and traditional (*ilobola*/dowry)	1 358	8.6	7.1–10.3
Married, civil and religious	1 931	7.6	6.2–9.2
Single, never married	4 589	22.9	21.5–24.4
Married, but separated	174	12.0	7.7–18.2
Divorced	967	11.2	9.0–13.9
Living together, but not married	95	12.2	6.5–21.9
Widow/widower	663	18.8	15.4–22.6
Other	24	14.7	5.5–33.5

Source: Shisana et al. 2005

prevalence among educators is highest for those aged 25–34 (21.4 per cent), followed by those aged 35–44 (12.8 per cent). Older educators (55 years and older) had the lowest HIV prevalence (3.1 per cent).

The findings also indicate that the highest HIV prevalence was among educators who were single (22.9 per cent) and major racial differences in HIV prevalence were observed. Black educators had a prevalence of 16.3 per cent, compared to whites, coloureds and Asians who had a combined prevalence of less than 1 per cent. Young black female educators (18–24 years old) had a much higher HIV prevalence of 17.4 per cent, compared with 12 per cent among their male counterparts. The sex differences widened substantially for black educators aged 25–29, where women had a prevalence of 30.4 per cent, in contrast with 14.5 per cent among men in the same age group (see Figure 5.1).

Among women educators, HIV prevalence peaked at 25–29 years old (29.2 per cent), thereafter declining rapidly to 17.5 per cent at ages 35–39. HIV prevalence among women continued to decline rapidly, until reaching a low of 5.2 per cent among women educators aged 50-54.

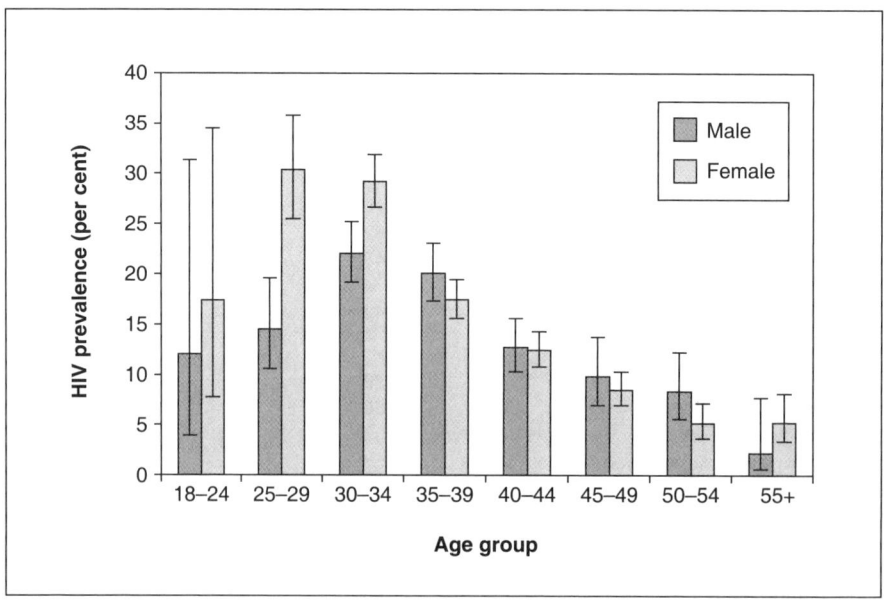

Figure 5.1 HIV prevalence by age and sex among 12 022 black South African educators from the ELRC/HSRC survey, 2004.

Source: Shisana et al. 2005

Table 5.2 Overall HIV prevalence among educators in the ELRC/HSRC survey by province, South Africa, 2004.

Province	Number surveyed	HIV-positive (per cent)	95 per cent CI
Western Cape	2 134	1.1	0.6–2.0
Eastern Cape	1 855	13.8	12.0–15.8
Northern Cape	891	4.3	2.9–6.5
Free State	1 152	12.4	10.1–15.0
KwaZulu-Natal	3 627	21.8	19.8–23.9
North West	1 437	10.4	8.7–12.4
Gauteng	2 772	6.4	5.4–7.7
Mpumalanga	1 315	19.1	16.2–22.3
Limpopo	1 905	8.6	7.3–10.1

Source: Shisana et al. 2005

The curve for men rose slowly from 12 per cent among those aged 18–24 to 14.5 per cent among those aged 25–29. It then rose very sharply, reaching a peak at 22.1 per cent among men aged 30–34; thereafter it remained high at 20 per cent among men aged 35–39. It then declined rapidly to a low of 2.2 per cent among men aged 55 years and older.

Educators working in schools located in urban formal settlements had a significantly lower HIV prevalence (6.3 per cent) than those working in urban informal settlements (13.9 per cent) and rural areas (16.8 per cent).

The study also investigated the HIV prevalence of educators by the province in which they were teaching and found significant differences. Educators employed in KwaZulu-Natal and Mpumalanga had the highest HIV prevalence (more than 19 per cent), compared with the other provinces (see Table 5.2). The second group of provinces with high HIV prevalence (more than 10 per cent, but less than 19 per cent) were the Eastern Cape, Free State and North West. The provinces with HIV prevalence under 10 per cent were Limpopo, Gauteng, Northern Cape and Western Cape, which had the lowest HIV prevalence at 1.1 per cent.

In relation to socio-economic status, HIV prevalence varied. Results showed that educators with a first degree at tertiary level, or higher, had the lowest HIV prevalence (10 per cent). Those with a lower level of formal education, for example, Grade 12 or lower, had a prevalence of 13.9 per cent. The prevalence was, however, not significantly lower than among those surveyed who held diplomas or an occupational certificate (15.9 per cent).

HIV prevalence by income of educators showed statistically significant differences; those with low income (below R60 000) had the highest HIV prevalence of 17.5 per cent; those with medium income (R60 000–R132 000) had an HIV prevalence of 12.1 per cent, while those with high income (more than R132 000) had the lowest HIV prevalence at 5.4 per cent. Educators who reported that they do not have money for basics like food and clothes had the highest HIV prevalence, compared to those who reported to have most of these necessities, but few luxury goods. HIV prevalence among this more economically vulnerable group was even higher when compared with rates among educators who had enough money for extra, non-essential goods.

The prevalence of HIV was highest among educators working in combined primary and secondary schools (16.5 per cent) (see Table 5.3). There was also a high prevalence of slightly more than 12 per cent at primary and secondary school sites. Less experienced educators were seen to be more likely to be HIV-positive. Those with less than four years' experience had an HIV prevalence of 21.1 per cent; those with five to nine years' experience had an HIV prevalence of 19.5 per cent, but

Table 5.3 Overall HIV prevalence by type of educational institution, position in educational system and years of teaching experience in the ELRC/HSRC survey, South Africa, 2004.

	Number surveyed	HIV-positive (percentage)	95 per cent CI
Type of institution			
Primary school	9 528	12.3	11.4–13.3
Combined	1 447	16.5	13.7–19.7
Secondary/high school	6 006	12.5	11.2–14.0
Position in educational system			
Educator	12 669	14.1	13.2–15.0
Senior educator	1 846	9.6	8.1–11.4
Education specialist	534	10.0	7.5–13.1
Deputy-principal/principal	1 709	7.3	6.0–8.8
Years of teaching experience			
0–4	2 031	21.1	19.1–23.3
5–9	2 724	19.5	17.8–21.4
10–14	4 484	14.8	13.5–16.2
15–19	2 712	8.8	7.6–10.2
20–24	2 416	7.0	5.9–8.3
25–29	1 494	5.4	4.1–7.1
30+	1 105	2.6	1.8–3.8

Source: Shisana et al. 2005

those with fifteen years' or more experience had a prevalence of less than 9 per cent. Therefore the most experienced educators were less likely to be living with HIV.

In Table 5.4, we see that most of the educators in the sample were teaching Foundation Phase, as well as Foundation Languages. Another large group of educators were Mathematics educators followed by Economics and Management. The HIV epidemic has left almost no learning area untouched. Other than the observation that HIV prevalence was high in all groups, except among Technology educators, it was found to be highest among Mathematics and Science educators at 12.9 per cent and 12.6 per cent respectively. It was also revealing that there was high HIV prevalence among those teaching general subjects, whose ranks are mostly comprised of black educators. However, it was also striking to learn that of all the subjects/learning areas, educators teaching Additional Languages had the highest HIV prevalence (23 per cent). Further analysis indicates that this group is comprised of black educators mostly teaching Portuguese in KwaZulu-Natal. Given that, as indicated earlier, there is a shortage of educators in certain subject areas, this is already a cause for a concern.

Table 5.4 Teachers in the ELRC/HSRC survey: HIV prevalence by learning area taught (trained in), South Africa, 2004.

Learning areas	Number surveyed	HIV-positive (percentage)	95 per cent CI
Foundation Phase	10 552	12.9	11.6–14.2
Foundation Languages	9 922	11.2	10.0–12.6
Additional Languages	1 086	23.6	19.2–28.7
Arts and Culture	2 777	13.2	9.7–17.6
Economics and Management Sciences	4 059	14.1	11.7–16.9
Social Sciences	2 255	11.8	9.3–15.0
Life Orientation	8 814	13.4	11.4–15.7
Mathematics	6 129	12.9	11.5–14.4
Natural Sciences	5 752	12.6	10.3–15.2
Technology	5 429	7.4	4.7–11.7
Special	59	0.0	–
Other	233	13.8	11.9–16.1

Source: Shisana et al. 2005

Determinants of HIV/AIDS

Most educators in this study reported having one current sexual partner. About 10 per cent of black educators reported having had two or more sexual partners in the past year, followed by 4 per cent of the coloured population. When data were disaggregated by the race and sex of the educator, it is evident that a significant proportion of male educators – in contrast to female educators – had multiple partners, which is a risk factor for sexually transmitted infections (STIs) and HIV/AIDS. Previous to providing a sample specimen for HIV testing for this survey, a large proportion of educators had had an HIV test (57.4 per cent), and of these, 92.6 per cent were told the results of their test. Notably, of those 57.4 per cent who had had an HIV test, 90.9 per cent were HIV-positive. Finally, 58.9 per cent of educators who knew prior to this study that they were HIV-positive used a condom with their regular partner at last sexual intercourse.

The majority of respondents (94.7 per cent males and 95.9 per cent females) knew that HIV could not be transmitted through using eating utensils used by someone with AIDS. With regard to the so-called 'virgin myth', the majority of educators (males, 96.5 per cent and females, 96.4 per cent) did not believe that having sex with a virgin could cure HIV. However there was a small number of educators who believed this myth (1.9 per cent males and 2.2 per cent females). The respondents were also mostly aware of behaviours that increase the risk of infection. Only around 8 per cent of both male and female respondents did not know that HIV could be transmitted through anal sex with an HIV-positive person. The majority of respondents knew that a person could look healthy while they have HIV (95.5 per cent males and 95.0 per cent females). They also knew that one could protect oneself from HIV by using condoms correctly each time one had sex (95.6 per cent males and 95.7 per cent females). Most respondents were aware that HIV could be transmitted through contact with infected blood (98.6 per cent of males and 98.7 per cent of females).

Of those surveyed, 15.9 per cent of males and 17.7 per cent of females believed that HIV could be spread through sneezing. On the question of HIV being transmitted through oral sex, there were a few respondents who said they did not know (16.3 per cent males and 15.6 per cent females). A fairly small percentage responded false to this statement (11.1 per cent males and 7 per cent females) and 72.4 per cent males and 77.3 per cent females said it was true that HIV could be transmitted through oral sex. A small number of respondents did not know that HIV could be transmitted through breastfeeding (11.6 per cent of males and 8.8 per cent of females), compared to 8.8 per cent of males and 6.3 per cent of females who responded false to this question. There were more educators (79.5 per cent males and 84.8 per cent females) who knew about mother-to-child HIV transmission risk associated with breastfeeding. Finally, in relation to antiretroviral medicines (ARVs), the majority of the educators (83.7 per cent males and 82.3 per cent females) knew that once one was on ARVs, one would have to take them forever, compared to 2.8 per cent males and 2.2 per cent females who responded false. Compared to the group who responded false, the percentage of those who did not know was higher (13.4 per cent males and 15.4 per cent females).

The study also looked at age mixing of educators, especially those educators who had partners either ten years younger or older than themselves. It was found that 14.1 per cent of male educators had a partner who was ten years younger than themselves, while only 0.55 per cent of women had a partner who was ten years younger than themselves. This suggests that more older men tend to have sex with much younger women. In comparing this finding to HIV prevalence, it was found that among male educators, those with partners younger than them by ten years or more were more likely to be HIV-positive, compared to those male educators whose partners were older than they were by ten years or more (16.5 per cent and 9.7 per cent).

Mobility and HIV

Among those surveyed, public educators residing in rural areas and those working in rural schools had significantly higher HIV prevalence than public educators residing in urban areas and teaching in urban schools (see Table 5.5). Public educators whose residence was further than ten kilometres away from home also had a slightly higher HIV prevalence rate (13.5 per cent) than public educators who travelled less than ten kilometres to their school (12.2 per cent), but the differences are not significant.

Migration after completion of training, in particular to a rural area, has been associated with higher HIV prevalence. HIV rates were lower among individuals who took up a post in the same area as close family. By mapping patterns of migration after 1994, it was revealed that an educator who moves with his/her family is less likely to contract HIV than an educator who is forced to leave his/her family behind (see Table 5.6).

Table 5.5 Residence area and HIV status of South African public educators in the ELRC/HSRC survey, 2004.

Educators' residence area	HIV-positive		
	Number surveyed	Percentage	95 per cent CI
Geolocality of residence			
Urban	933	9.7	8.9–10.6
Rural	1 111	16.9	15.8–18.0
Geolocality of school			
Urban formal	421	6.3	5.4–7.4
Urban informal	155	13.9	11.5–16.6
Rural	1 464	16.8	15.8–17.8
Distance from residence to school			
Near (within 10 km)	1 130	12.2	11.3–13.1
Far (more than 10 km)	917	13.5	12.5–14.6

Source: Shisana et al. 2005

Table 5.6 Migration and HIV status of educators in the ELRC/HSRC survey, South Africa, 2004.

Migration status of educators	HIV-positive		
	Number surveyed	Percentage	95 per cent CI
In first move since 1994			
Family moved with me	102	10.4	8.4–12.8
Family stayed behind	161	15.2	12.8–17.8
No family, on my own at the time	93	15.2	12.3–18.7
In second move since 1994			
Family moved with me	30	6.6	4.5–9.8
Family stayed behind	95	15.6	12.7–19.2
No family, on my own at the time	32	10.7	7.5–15.0
In third move since 1994			
Family moved with me	36	6.5	4.6–9.1
Family stayed behind	79	15.4	12.2–19.2
No family, on my own at the time	19	11.5	7.4–17.6
In most recent move since 1994			
Family moved with me	17	4.5	2.3–7.5
Family stayed behind	43	12.9	9.4–17.5
No family, on my own at the time	11	10.7	5.6–19.5

Source: Shisana et al. 2005

Table 5.7 Mobility and HIV status of educators in the ELRC/HSRC survey, South Africa, 2004.

Mobility levels of educators	HIV-positive		
	Number surveyed	Percentage	95 per cent CI
In past 12 months been away from home for more than one month			
Yes	328	17.8	15.8–20.0
No	1 710	12.1	11.4–12.9
Number of nights per week usually stay away from home			
None	203	8.6	7.2–10.4
1–2 nights	77	16.5	12.8–21.0
3–4 nights	87	16.7	13.5–20.5
5 nights	122	20.5	19.9–24.7
6 and more nights	107	27.6	23.0–32.7

Source: Shisana et al. 2005

The study results clearly suggest that mobility is strongly associated with increased risk of HIV among educators. Table 5.7 shows that having stayed away from home for more than one month in the past twelve months is significantly associated with HIV. Educators who do not sleep out of their family homes had the lowest HIV prevalence (8.6 per cent), while those who stay away one or two nights per week have about twice the risk (16.5 per cent) of HIV infection.

Findings of the ELRC/HRSC study: Student educators
Demographic characteristics of student educators
The study examined the demographic characteristics of student educators (see Table 5.8). The data are presented for: (1) combined third- and fourth-year education students; (2) third-year education students; and (3) fourth-year education students separately. Overall, the student educators were predominantly female.

Although black people comprise 79 per cent of the South African population and 77.4 per cent of the educators in the educator school survey, only 60 per cent of student educators in the student survey at contact universities were black and 30 per cent were white. The majority of student educators, as expected, were between 18 and 24 years old; these are the ages when newly graduated high school students enter tertiary institutions to pursue a career. Some of the students aged 25 and older were employed as educators and at the time of the study were upgrading their educational qualifications. The majority of these students were single, not married

Table 5.8 Demographic characteristics of the ELRC/HSRC sample of 1 056 student educators, South Africa, 2004.

Demographics	3rd and 4th years		3rd years		4th years	
	Number surveyed	%	N	%	N	%
Sex						
Male	351	33.4	305	33.7	46	31.3
Female	701	66.6	600	66.3	101	68.7
Race						
Black	631	59.9	526	58.0	105	71.9
White	312	29.6	288	31.8	24	16.4
Coloured	82	7.8	70	7.7	12	8.2
Indian/Asian	28	2.7	23	2.5	5	3.4
Age in years						
18–24	618	47.9	566	62.3	52	35.4
25–29	296	22.9	201	22.1	95	64.6
30–34	85	6.6	85	9.4	–	–
35+*	56	4.3	56	6.2	–	–
Current marital status						
Ever married	160	14.1	132	14.5	28	19.2
Never married	895	79.0	777	85.5	118	80.8
Economic status						
Not enough money for basics	122	11.7	97	10.8	25	17.2
Have money for food and clothes	382	36.7	307	34.3	75	51.7
Have most of the things	339	32.6	303	33.8	36	24.8
Some money for extra things	198	19.0	189	21.1	9	6.2

* 3rd years include age range of 18–54
* 4th years defined as < 30

Source: Shisana et al. 2005

and came from urban areas. The smallest proportion came from poor households, followed by those who came from households who meet the basic needs, but have very little left after buying food. One in five students came from households that are well provided with resources.

The socio-demographic analysis of the student educator sample suggests that the population of students entering the teaching profession is unlikely to remain in poor, under-resourced rural areas. Only a few white educators (8.5 per cent) were found in rural schools, as opposed to 91.5 per cent in urban schools, while 69.5 per cent of black educators were teaching at rural schools. Black student educators are likely to come from urban areas and they are the ones who are likely to be deployed to a school in a rural area. This presents challenges given that mobility and deployment to rural areas is associated with higher HIV prevalence (Shisana et al. 2005, xvii).

HIV status of education students

There are few reliable statistics on the HIV status of tertiary students in South Africa. The few studies that exist, including this one, have major limitations. The principal limitation is representativeness of the study population. For this reason, in studying educators, it is critical to estimate the percentage of HIV-positive students who are studying to be educators. Higher HIV prevalence is likely to mean higher death rates and fewer numbers of new educators available in the system. Table 5.9 shows HIV prevalence among 902 students studying to become educators.

Table 5.9 HIV prevalence among educators and education students, ELRC/HSRC survey, South Africa, 2004.

	Educators			Students		
	Number surveyed	Per cent HIV+	95 per cent CI	Number surveyed	Per cent HIV+	95 per cent CI
Demographics	17 088	12.7	12.0–13.5	902	8.2	6.6–10.2
Sex						
Male	5 455	12.7	11.6–13.9	291	4.8	2.9–8.0
Female	11 621	12.8	2.0–13.6	607	9.9	7.8–12.5
Race						
Black	12 022	16.3	15.5–17.1	546	13.2	10.6–16.3
White, coloured,						
Indian/Asian	5 007	0.6	0.4–0.9	354	0.6	0.1–2.2
Age in years						
18–24	240	6.5	3.4–12.1	528	4.4	2.9–6.5
25–34	4 282	21.4	19.8–23.1	327	14.7	11.2–19.0
35+	12 559	9.9	9.2–10.6	46	6.5	2.1–18.4
Household economic situation						
Not enough money/ money for food	9 841	14.8	13.9–15.7	426	13.1	10.3–16.7
Have most important things/extras	7 130	9.5	8.5–10.6	465	3.7	2.3–5.8

Source: Shisana et al. 2005

Of the student educators tested in this study, 8.2 per cent were found to be HIV-positive. Third-year students were less likely to be HIV-positive (7 per cent) than the fourth-year students, whose prevalence was 15.5 per cent. Because the sample size of third- and fourth-year students was small, the two groups were combined. The HIV test results showed that females had a much higher HIV prevalence (9.9 per cent) than males (4.8 per cent). Black students had a prevalence of 13.2 per cent, compared with coloureds, Indian/Asians and whites combined, whose HIV prevalence was less than 1 per cent.

Examining the HIV distribution by age revealed that HIV prevalence was highest for those aged 25–29 years. Married students had a much higher HIV prevalence, compared with single students, but this might be confounded by age, given that the majority of educators were younger and they had lower HIV prevalence. When the relationship between HIV prevalence and marital status is examined for each age group separately, the differences disappear, except for 18–24-year-olds, which is the largest age group (59 per cent). However, relatively few are married (6 per cent), so the estimates may be unreliable and no statistically significant differences were found.

Given evidence that socio-economic status is related to HIV among educators in South Africa, it was necessary for this relationship to be assessed in the student population. The results indicated that socio-economic status was associated with HIV status; those with perceived low socio-economic status had a much higher HIV prevalence (13.1 per cent) than those with perceived higher status (3.7 per cent).

The findings on HIV prevalence require further discussion. The 8 per cent HIV prevalence seems to be lower than the findings cited by Labby Ramrathan, who quotes a prevalence of 22.9 per cent among students at the University of Durban-Westville (2003). However, these are not strictly comparable groups. The University of Durban-Westville students were drawn from a convenience sample, largely of black African origin. The 8 per cent is also not comparable to the 1.1 per cent observed HIV prevalence among students at Rand Afrikaans University (RAU, now called the University of Johannesburg), which was then 30 per cent African; 50 per cent white; 11 per cent Indian/Asian and 8.8 per cent coloured (Centre for Sociological Research 2002). The latter study used a purposive sample and has a different racial profile. Even the authors agree that the true prevalence in this group is likely to be much higher. At this time, there is not a student population against which the HIV results in the current study can be compared.

The observed prevalence of 8 per cent among these student educators should be a source of concern. Although the sample may not be representative of third- and fourth-year education students in tertiary institutions, the observed prevalence of 8 per cent is quite high for people who are being trained to enter the teaching profession. Certainly, they contribute to higher HIV prevalence among educators, even though educators may independently have a high HIV prevalence.

Factors contributing to HIV/AIDS infections in student educators

We found that nearly two-thirds of students were sexually active, making them vulnerable to STIs, including HIV. The risky sexual behaviour examined was multiple partners and condom use. Other factors such as age mixing are not reported because there were too many missing values, suggesting that the results may not be reliable. The results were interesting: 35.6 per cent were abstinent, but nearly 12 per cent of students reported multiple partners in the past twelve months. A fairly high percentage of students reported condom use during their last sexual contact with a regular partner (65.9 per cent) and even more with a non-regular partner (83.2 per cent). These findings are similar to other studies among university students. Among black South African university students, men reported a mean of 2.7 and women 1.2 sexual partners in the past twelve months. Two-thirds (66 per cent) of both female and male university students reported consistently (always) using a condom during sexual intercourse in the past four weeks (Peltzer et al. 2005). A study at RAU found that 74.2 per cent of sexually active South African university students from RAU had used a condom during their last sexual encounter, but also that 43.5 per cent had engaged in casual sex in the past twelve months (Centre for Sociological Research 2002).

Conclusions

HIV/AIDS is said not to discriminate against age or race, but there seems to be complacency in relation to condom use among individuals of certain age and race groups. This study found that generally younger male and female respondents used condoms more regularly than their older counterparts. Being HIV-positive was associated with consistent condom use with a regular sex partner. However, condoms were not consistently used during sexual acts with non-regular partners. This latter phenomenon is cause for concern. Knowledge of HIV/AIDS and perceived threat of HIV infection showed small associations with condom use, which is consistent with other research (see, for example, Camlin and Chimbwete 2003; Sheeran, Abraham and Orbell 1999). HIV risk perception was only associated with consistent condom use with a regular and not with a non-regular partner.

This study found that educators residing in rural areas and those working in rural schools had higher HIV prevalence than educators residing in urban areas and teaching in urban schools. A possible explanation for this is that teachers in poorer rural areas fall in the high-income group by local standards, possibly resulting in them being seen as a desirable group with whom to have a sexual relationship. This suggests that income may be an additional risk factor. For example, higher income earners are able to buy sex and alcohol. This risk factor suggests that affluent groups in a society may be at risk because of their ability not only to buy luxuries, but also to attract multiple sexual partners (Shisana et al. 2003).

Student educators are the future of the education system, but unfortunately, 8.2 per cent of those students tested were HIV-positive. Moreover, educators are desperately needed in South Africa's rural areas, yet students seem to be trained for urban schools. These findings lead to a number of conclusions, which require specific HIV/AIDS policy interventions in the education sector:

- Women were the majority – 68 per cent – of educators in the education sector. When the review of the findings was restricted to women and men aged 25–34 years, women had higher HIV prevalence. Unabated infection among this important group will impact on the pool of educators. This means that there should be more effort to empower female teachers. Gender imbalances should also be addressed by creating a social environment that discourages men from engaging in risky behaviour that puts them – and consequently women – at risk of HIV.
- When compared to other groups, HIV disproportionately affects black teachers. Interventions should target this group, which had an average lower socio-economic status than other groups, and where HIV prevalence was concentrated in the high-risk age group of 25–34.
- HIV prevalence varied by province, indicating higher levels in KwaZulu-Natal and Mpumalanga, which had the highest HIV prevalence (more than 19 per cent) compared to the others. Heavily impacted provinces need to be targeted with interventions and the requisite resources to cope with the impact of HIV/AIDS.

- All educators should receive training on HIV/AIDS, aimed at reducing risky behaviour, such as age mixing, lack of condom use and multiple partners. These risky behaviours unfold in various ways: men reported having had more multiple partnerships than women; males who had a sexual partner ten years younger than themselves were more likely to be infected with HIV and older people were less likely to use condoms.
- In order to address these risky behaviours, educators – who are a 'captive audience' – should be exposed to HIV prevention programmes that address issues of serial monogamy, concurrent sexual partnerships, having sexual partners within one's age group and the importance of HIV testing.
- Policies should facilitate an increase in regular family visits; the moving of family members with public educators to teaching posts and the provision of housing for educators nearer to schools. Provinces and districts with higher HIV prevalence should be urgently targeted. Existing priorities do seem to address these geographic locations, but programmes designed in partnership with the Department of Education, national unions and schools need to develop tools to give educators skills to negotiate safer sex, especially young, recently qualified educators in these areas.
- Initiatives could be implemented to attract educators to remote and rural schools. Possible initiatives would provide financial support to student educators who wish to do their teaching practice in government rural schools in the district in which they hope to work the following year. However, teachers working in remote areas must also be supported in migrating with their families. This support should include assistance with travel costs, living expenses for the duration of the teaching practice and a rural teaching service package, with extra benefits in terms of housing, locality allowance and permanent employment.

This chapter has provided an overview of the level of HIV prevalence in South Africa's education sector. It is a modest contribution to the literature on the impact of HIV/AIDS on society. The education sector remains severely under-resourced in various ways. The South African Department of Education and the national unions, together with civil society must address the sector's needs for qualified, motivated and healthy teachers. HIV/AIDS threatens to make this objective more difficult, as it affects the most vulnerable in our schools.

Note

1. This chapter is based on Shisana et al. (2005) and was written with contributions from Shandir Ramlagan, Olive Shisana, Cathy Connolly and Khangelani Zuma.

References

Badcock-Walters, Peter and Marelize Görgens. 2001. *HIV/AIDS Impact on Education in Africa: An Analysis of Conferences, Workshops, Seminars, Meetings and Summits Focusing on HIV/AIDS Impact on Education in Africa – December 1999 to June 2001*. Durban: HEARD (Health Economics and HIV/AIDS Research Division).

Bennell, Paul. 2003. 'The Impact of the AIDS Epidemic on Schooling in Sub-Saharan Africa'. Background paper from the Association for the Development of Education in Africa (ADEA) biennial meeting, December. Available at http://www.adeanet.org/biennial2003/papers/10A_AIDS%20Benell_ENG_final.pdf, accessed 17 December 2007.

Camlin, Carol and Chiweni Chimbwete. 2003. 'Does Knowing Someone with AIDS Affect Condom Use? An Analysis from South Africa'. *AIDS Education and Prevention* 15(3), June: 231–44.

CCR (Centre for Conflict Resolution). 2006. 'HIV/AIDS and Human Security in South Africa'. Unpublished concept paper for the seminar 'HIV/AIDS and Human Security in South Africa', Cape Town, 26-27 June.

Centre for Sociological Research. 2002. *HIV/AIDS and Students at RAU: Final Report*. Johannesburg: Centre for Sociological Research.

Coombe, Carol. 2002. 'Managing the Impact of HIV/AIDS on the Education Sector, 2000'. Available at http://www.hivaidsclearinghouse.unesco.org/ev_en.php?ID=1250_201&ID2=DO_TOPIC, accessed 15 December 2004.

Kelly, Michael J. 2000. *Planning for Education in the Context of HIV/AIDS*. Paris: UNESCO.

Peltzer, Karl, Olive Shisana, Eric Udjo, David Wilson, Thomas Rehle, Cathy Connolly, Khangelani Zuma, Lebo Letlape, Julia Louw, Leickness Simbayi, Nompumelelo Zungu-Dirwayi, Shandir Ramlagan, Kgobati Magome, Elsie Hall and Makola Phurutse. 2005. *Educator Supply and Demand in the South African Public Education System: Integrated Report*. Cape Town: Human Sciences Research Council Press.

Ramrathan, Labby. 2003. 'Troubling the Numbers: Is Teacher Demand Projection Possible within the Context of HIV/AIDS?' *South African Journal of Higher Education* 17(2): 177–86.

SADTU (South African Democratic Teachers' Union). 2003. 'HIV/AIDS and Public Education in South Africa: Focal Points for a Research Agenda'. Discussion paper.

Sheeran, Paschal, Charles Abraham and Sheina Orbell. 1999. 'Psychosocial Correlates of Heterosexual Condom Use: A Meta-Analysis'. *Psychological Bulletin* 125(1): 90–131.

Shisana, Olive, Karl Peltzer, Nompumelelo Zungu-Dirwayi and Julia Louw. 2005. *The Health of Our Educators: A Focus on HIV/AIDS in South African Public Schools*. Cape Town: Human Sciences Research Council Press.

Shisana, Olive, Nompumelelo Zungu-Dirwayi, Leickness Simbayi and Yoesrie Toefy. 2003. 'Marital Status and the Risk of HIV Infection in South Africa'. Paper presented at the South African AIDS Conference, Durban, August.

UNICEF (United Nations (International) Children's (Emergency) Fund). 1999. *Children Orphaned by AIDS: Front-Line Responses from Eastern and Southern Africa.* New York: UNICEF.

6

Rural Livelihoods and Land

——•——

Ruth Hall

Introduction

In the rural areas of southern Africa, there is an urgent need to understand and respond to the effects of HIV/AIDS. Research shows that these effects include the disruption of migration patterns and the remittance economy on which many rural households depend, as well as a loss of cash income and assets. HIV also increases dependence on subsistence agricultural production for household food and reduces the cash and labour needed to support farming. The virus's influence extends to increased conflict over land rights and inheritance.

The epidemic has already had a severe impact on the land rights and livelihoods of people living in the two distinct rural sectors that characterise the southern African region: communal areas under tribal authority and privately owned commercial farms. This chapter reviews what is known about the interaction of HIV/AIDS and the already tenuous economies of poor households in these two sectors. It explores whether, in the livelihoods of rural households, HIV/AIDS is 'a shock like any other' (Baylies 2002), or whether it differs from others both qualitatively and in its severity, and considers the implications for survival and recovery.

There is a growing body of literature on the impact of HIV/AIDS on rural livelihoods in southern Africa – on the assets, incomes and livelihood strategies of rural households, and therefore on agricultural production and food security. HIV/AIDS interacts with other trends that are also shaping the livelihoods of rural South Africans and southern Africans, such as the restructuring of the agricultural economy, reduced state support for agriculture, deregulation and job-shedding. This chapter focuses on the implications for securing land rights and land-based livelihoods among the poor and therefore the ways in which the coping strategies and practices of HIV-infected and -affected populations articulate with other processes and trends.

Such analysis requires distinguishing between presumptions (postulates) of the impact of HIV/AIDS and the available evidence. Much of the research data informing strategies by governments, subregional and international organisations are based either on national aggregated estimates (for example, prevalence data from antenatal clinics), or qualitative case studies (for example, biographies and narratives of individuals), which provide important information at the macro- and micro-levels. Much of the literature rests on a hypothesised chain of causality from individual illness and death to social (and economic) collapse. This may not assist in predicting the future or in informing intervention strategies and should be interrogated. More attention on the social dynamics of the epidemic is needed. A starting point for rural areas is to understand the role that property rights and land rights, in particular, play in underpinning human security.

HIV/AIDS in the context of rural livelihoods

In effect, HIV/AIDS tends to exacerbate existing development problems through its catalytic effects and systemic impact (Topouzis 1998, 1). In southern African countries, agriculture is the mainstay of up to 80 per cent of the population (ILO 2004). In the subsistence sector, food production for household consumption is predominantly dependent on women's labour (ILO 2004, 26). Rural households tend to rely on agricultural production for a portion of their consumption needs and to sell a portion of their produce, in order to generate some cash income, but agricultural production by the poor is usually one of a number of livelihood strategies, including waged labour and small businesses. Colonial (and apartheid) policies of reserves and influx control established a pattern of oscillating migrancy from the rural areas to urban factories and mines as a central pillar of rural livelihoods, providing a crucial stream of remittance income in rural households. Where other sources of income have ceased or are under threat, households may invest more of their savings and effort in agricultural production.

Relative to other sectors of the economy, agriculture is disproportionately severely affected by the HIV epidemic (Jayne et al. 2005). This is *not* due to higher HIV prevalence in rural areas – indeed, prevalence is generally higher in urban areas, even though it is probable that in absolute numbers, rural infections outnumber urban (Topouzis 1998), but rather due to the more limited capacity of the rural population to absorb shock and to withstand the loss of incomes and labour (De Waal and Tumushabe 2003). An assessment of the impact of HIV/AIDS on vulnerability to food insecurity in Malawi, Zambia and Zimbabwe confirms that affected rural households are more vulnerable to food insecurity (SADC FANR 2003).

Declining agricultural production

In the rural areas of southern Africa, there is a declining life expectancy and increased food insecurity, which suggests that the Millennium Development Goals (MDGs) will not be met (ILO 2004, 26). The first and most obvious impact of the epidemic has been declining production in agriculture, particularly smallholder farming, which is the predominant occupation of rural people in southern Africa. Research in Zambia showed that households in which the household head had died of AIDS reduced the area they cultivated by an average of 53 per cent (ILO 2004, 25). The loss of some family members and the sickness of others also sometimes prevent smallholders from harvesting and selling cash crops (ILO 2004, 24).

Another observed trend is the reduction in marketed surplus, as production declines and a larger proportion of produce is consumed (IRRD 2002). For example, Mphale, Rwambali and Makoae observed a reduction in cash and non-cash incomes among small-scale farmers in Lesotho (2002). These dynamics are shaped by the average of two years of adult household members' labour lost between the onset of AIDS-related illness and death.

Women are predominantly responsible for food production for household consumption in southern Africa and the burden of caring for sick household members also falls on women, greatly reducing available agricultural labour (ILO 2004, 24–26; Action Aid 2006). The impacts of HIV/AIDS on rural livelihoods are thus gendered and the burdens of the epidemic may exacerbate gender inequalities (Mutangadura 2005). Time allocation studies also reveal the gendered burden of the epidemic on rural households. As women's days are spent fetching water, preparing food and caring for the sick, there is less time to perform the tasks that sustain life, such as cultivating crops, or earning a small income. A study in South Africa, for instance, showed that in almost half the households surveyed, the primary caregiver for an AIDS patient had taken time off from formal or informal employment, or from schooling. Women and girls may lose as much as 60 per cent of time from other housework or cultivation tasks, affecting the ability of poor households to grow food for consumption or sale (Heyzer 2004).

Declining crop yields are also the result of insufficient inputs, such as fertilisers, seed and labour. As well as lower yields, AIDS-affected households reduce the range of crops produced, usually focusing on food crops for household consumption, rather than cash crops for sale (Tibbo and Drimie 2006). Alongside cultivation and non-farm economic activities, livestock constitute an important store of wealth, providing a buffer against destitution. Livestock is an easily liquidated asset and so households in distress often sell animals to pay for food, medicines and funerals, once other sources of income have dried up (Drimie and Gandure 2005, 15; Mphale, Rwambali and Makoae 2002). HIV/AIDS leads households to sell assets for consumption purposes and to pay medical expenses, and this decline in resources reduces households' productive and reproductive capabilities, leading in extreme cases to 'utter destitution and household dissolution' (De Waal and Tumushabe 2003, 3).

Country-level studies have confirmed that these impacts are similar across the southern African region. The loss of regular income from the employment of a household member was the first and most salient impact. The studies, conducted in Kenya, Lesotho and South Africa, and a similar study by the Oxford Committee for Famine Relief (OXFAM) in Malawi, converged in finding that the main impacts of HIV/AIDS on rural households were:

- loss of income due to the loss of a job, or an inability to work due to illness, or the burden of caring for the ill;
- depletion of savings and sale of assets to meet medical expenses and to pay for funerals;
- limitation of livelihood options as a result of chronic illness, with land use assuming greater importance as a result;
- reduced capacity to use the land as a result of illness and caring for the ill, sale of livestock and inability to purchase agricultural inputs; and
- vulnerability to loss of land following AIDS-related deaths. This resulted from a lack of secure tenure for widows and orphans. (FAO and SARPN 2002, 3)

In a number of studies in southern and eastern Africa, common responses to the chronic illness of an adult family member, and particularly the household head, or main income earner, were distress sales of land, implements and other household assets, and property-grabbing by extended families and neighbours from widows and orphans and vulnerable children (OVC) (Drimie and Gandure 2005; IRRD 2002; IRIN-News 2005; Izumi 2006a, 2006b). Further themes emerging from the literature are asset-stripping and theft; ratcheting down assets for consumption; rising indebtedness and a diminished ability to manage debt; terminating cultivation, or reducing the area of land cultivated, or the period of the year in which it is cultivated; leasing out or selling land rights in informal property markets; and vulnerability to losing informal land rights. Furthermore, the literature tells us consistently that the decline in food production and nutrition in turn precipitates AIDS-related deaths.

A study conducted for the Human Sciences Research Council (HSRC) in KwaZulu-Natal illustrates the impact of lost income on agricultural production and the livelihoods of the poor (IRRD 2002, 81). Among the many household-level case studies, the story of Bongi C. is emblematic of many others. The death of her son, who had been a breadwinner, hampered the efforts of Bongi, an elderly widow, to cultivate vegetables to sustain a growing extended family across three generations. Following his death and the loss of his income, she found herself unable to continue to buy fertiliser, to hire a tractor, or to maintain the fencing around her plot. For this reason, her production diminished from two harvests per year to one, greatly reducing her ability to meet household food needs.

In the long term, the agrarian economy will face substantial losses of its total labour force (employed and self-employed). Skills and indigenous knowledge of cultivation are being lost, as adults sicken and cannot teach their children traditional methods of cultivation and animal husbandry (Drimie and Gandure 2005).

Conflict over land rights

Country-level studies conducted under the auspices of the Food and Agricultural Organisation (FAO) found that the impact of the HIV/AIDS epidemic on households increased the need for land, but decreased the ability of households to use land effectively and rendered their hold on land more tenuous. This makes for an explosive combination. HIV/AIDS has been found to increase the incidence of land-related disputes, both among relatives and between relatives of the deceased and traditional authorities, or others with the power to allocate customary land (FAO and SARPN 2002). Exacerbated by HIV/AIDS, land-related conflicts revolve around inheritance and the ability of surviving household members to exclude others. The widespread practice of 'widow inheritance' (when a man is expected to marry his brother's widow) is reportedly on the decline, due to stigma and fears of infection, but what remains is an entrenched norm in patrilineal societies – that women cannot inherit.

Property-grabbing is often a punitive measure against widows, who are blamed for infecting their husbands with the virus, or for bringing about their deaths through witchcraft (Izumi 2006a).

The widows of men who have already died from AIDS no longer have land to grow the food that will keep them alive, because in many places single and widowed women are denied the right to own land and property in their own names. When combined with poverty and gender inequality, HIV/AIDS creates a deadly scenario for women and their families (Heyzer 2004).

There is not only land-grabbing 'from below', by other rural households, but also 'from above', by wealthier households, by local political and business elites and also by brokers for external commercial interests (Moyo and Hall 2007). Indeed, an outcome of increased sensitivity to shocks and declining resilience is increased inequality: 'some may even benefit from the impoverishment of others, for instance by obtaining access to land (through dispossessing dissolving households) or by hiring cheap labour' (De Waal and Tumushabe 2003, 4).

Paradoxically, alongside increased pressure on land, another observed trend in rural areas is abandonment of land, but also an increase in informal transactions in land rights, including informal leasing and informal sales of land held under customary tenure regimes (IRRD 2002). Sharecropping seems to be on the rise, as those who have land, but are unable to produce – particularly women-headed households – seek out the labour and investments of those who are landless, though they may fail to reassert control over their land and to reclaim it for their own use (Mphale, Rwambali and Makoae 2002).

Household formation

In rural households, as in urban areas, skipped-generation 'granny' households are on the rise, as are 'bloated' households, where extended families absorb not only children, but also vulnerable adults from other households. As in urban areas, there is a threshold beyond which households cease to absorb additional members and these conditions breed vulnerability to abuse, exploitation and violence (FAO News 2004; FAO-SAFR 2006). As in urban areas, there is increased reliance on social grants, though not necessarily the means (telecommunications, transport, access to identity documents) by which to access these. As in urban areas, the illness and death of income earners is exacerbated by the time and opportunity cost of home-based care, which takes other family members away from productive and income-earning activities.

Migration

Mobility and labour migration are recognised as vectors of HIV transmission, along with poverty, underdevelopment and gender inequalities (IOM 2004). Yet, just as the epidemic has spread because of the mobility of populations, new patterns of migration have emerged in response to it. Longitudinal studies and qualitative data demonstrate how the epidemic has disrupted migration patterns and the remittance economy on which many rural households, particularly within the former Bantustans or 'homelands', depend. The major new trend is the growth of 'reverse migration', as migrants to urban centres who have become ill return to extended family homes in rural areas to be cared for (SAMP 2004). These rural households experience a double burden of HIV/AIDS: they lose urban remittances from employed household members, while carrying extra medical expenses, the cost of caring for the ill and funeral expenses (Drimie and Gandure 2005).

Existing evidence suggests that the epidemic also leads to contracted patterns of migration arising from the declining ability of affected households to sustain jobs elsewhere, or to afford the high costs of transport. A study carried out under the auspices of the Southern African Development Community (SADC) found that HIV/AIDS leads to *decreased mobility* among affected rural households, which may affect their ability to access services and support, as well as cash income (SADC FANR 2003).

Coping strategies

Two paradigms present different ways of understanding the implications of HIV/AIDS for agrarian economies and rural livelihoods. Carolyn Baylies argues that HIV/AIDS is 'a shock like any other' to rural households dependent on land-based livelihoods and vulnerable to unpredictable changes in weather and market conditions (2002). This is not to say that the shock is not severe, but rather that there is no qualitative distinction between HIV/AIDS and other shocks that this population may experience, and thus that recovery will be shaped by established coping strategies that have been well documented historically, such as leasing out land, hiring out family labour, sale of livestock and other assets – short-term changes that enable a household to withstand a crisis and to recover over time.

An alternative perspective, proposed by Alex de Waal, is that the established literature on coping strategies is misplaced in the context of the epidemic. Instead, he argues, what we see is *a failure to cope*: strategies for survival that undermine the possibility of recovery (De Waal and Tumushabe 2003). In this view, HIV/AIDS is unlike other shocks because its effects are compounding and mutually reinforcing: implementing one of the short-term changes mentioned above often leads not to recovery, but to a downward spiral of increasing poverty. Counter-productive survival strategies inhibit recovery after the major shock of the loss of adult household members. Examples include the withdrawal of girls from school to provide domestic or income-generating labour and, at times, the wholesale disintegration of families and kinship networks (SADC FANR 2003). To drive his point home, De Waal claims that the convergence of HIV/AIDS and an episode of acute food insecurity produces 'new variant famine' (NVF), which, like a new virulent strain of a virus, is not susceptible to existing cures (De Waal and Tumushabe 2003, 1).

It is widely recognised that HIV-affected households are less able to deal with other external shocks (ILO 2004, 24–25). In addition, illness and death erode the traditional coping strategies and systems of mutual assistance among rural households. A study on vulnerability to food insecurity notes that the epidemic has led to marked reductions in agricultural production and income earning, and to earlier engagement in distress coping strategies, when rains fail, or other crisis conditions emerge (SADC FANR 2003). In the context of the epidemic, coping strategies pursued by rural households include: the rise of a range of tenancies, including sharecropping, as those most affected are less able to use the land they have; poor households developing a stronger preference for food crops over cash crops; and less sustainable natural resource use, as the allocation of time, labour and money changes when illness and death hit (FAO and SARPN 2002).

Farm worker communities on commercial farms
In southern Africa, family structures on commercial farms are marked by a more limited sense of community and are more restricted than in communal areas. Yet they face the same isolation from access to information, education, health and legal services, making them a segment of the population particularly vulnerable to HIV/AIDS (HRC 2003). The geographic isolation of commercial farms makes these people substantially insulated from state programmes that provide information and access to testing and services. A study conducted in Mpumalanga by the International Organisation for Migration (IOM), for instance, found that there was no means for farm workers on the twelve farms studied to obtain access to information on HIV/AIDS (2004, 10). Because of their isolation from the media and public infrastructure, specific measures are needed to target farm workers.

In some parts of the southern African region, a characteristic that makes farm workers more vulnerable to contracting HIV is the predominance of labour migration in rural labour markets. While farm workers are a stable population in some regions, elsewhere they are a mobile population, crossing borders, sometimes illegally, to secure work on farms. Some return periodically to their homes to remit incomes and maintain family ties. The widely recognised influx of Zimbabweans onto white commercial farms in Limpopo, the northernmost province of South Africa, is one such key area, but similar patterns have been observed in the western regions of Mozambique and the southern border area of Zambia. Like its rural-urban counterpart, oscillating migration splits up families, puts migrants and their spouses and boyfriends or girlfriends at risk of infection and fuels the perception that migrants bring the virus with them. Migrant farm workers, as a result, have been confronted with stigma and hostility from settled farm worker populations. However, the vulnerable condition of migrant farm workers is often overlooked in policy interventions.

The characteristics of farm worker communities do not only render them vulnerable to contracting HIV and isolated from support services. The comparatively reduced social networks of households affected by HIV-related deaths on commercial farms exacerbate the vulnerability of orphaned children and widowed women (Walker 2002). In particular, orphans on commercial farms are less likely than those in communal areas to have an extended family network to fall back on. They are less likely to be absorbed into other households and are more likely to constitute child-headed households. As the title of the only major study on HIV/AIDS on commercial farms in Zimbabwe suggests, orphans of farm workers often feel that 'we will bury ourselves' (Walker 2002). Even where jobs may be available, these orphans have been told they are not allowed to work because of laws prohibiting child labour (Walker 2002, 9). In response, the FAO in Zimbabwe has launched 'Junior Farmer Field Schools' to provide agricultural training to children orphaned by HIV/AIDS to enable them to produce food to survive.

Female farm workers, who are often not considered to be employees in their own right, are particularly vulnerable to losing both their jobs and their homes when their husbands or partners become ill or die (Izumi 2006a). Widows and orphans may be evicted from their homes, since access to housing on farms is usually part of an employment agreement between a landowner and male household head (Sunde and Kleinbooi 1999).

Table 6.1 Projected loss of agricultural labour force due to HIV/AIDS in southern Africa's most affected countries (2000–20).

Country	2000 (%)	2020 (%)
Botswana	6.6	23.2
Malawi	5.8	13.8
Mozambique	2.3	20.0
Namibia	3.0	26.0
South Africa	3.9	19.9
Tanzania	5.8	12.7
Zimbabwe	9.6	22.7

Source: FAO in ILO, 2004, 25

There is a high incidence of transactional sex among farm worker populations, a consequence of the dependence of women on relations with men, in order to secure access to employment on farms. This can lead to women entering into new relationships with permanent male workers, so as to secure their continued residence on farms and to negotiate continued employment – a factor that has also been blamed for the higher HIV prevalence on commercial farms than in surrounding areas in some countries (Izumi 2006a, 6). In addition, high levels of sexual abuse, which has been causally linked to alcohol and other substance abuse among farm workers, are thought to further increase the spread of HIV (IOM 2004, 12).

The FAO estimates that seven million agricultural workers died worldwide between 1985 and 2000 and in the most affected countries in sub-Saharan Africa, this accounted for up to 12.8 per cent of the total agricultural workforce (ILO 2004, 25). Studies in commercial agriculture in the SADC region have shown that some of the impacts of the epidemic contribute to the structural conditions that promote its spread, such as transactional sex (IOM 2004). Table 6.1 shows not the incidence of HIV/AIDS, but the proportion of the agricultural labour force lost (to illness or death) as a result of the epidemic, suggesting much higher rates of infection. The table illustrates variations between countries, but also the general trend that, over the coming decade or so, between one-fifth and one-quarter of the agricultural labour force will be lost to the epidemic in most countries in the SADC region.

In South Africa, the Agricultural Employers' Organisation (AEO) and agribusiness companies have warned that rates of absenteeism and deaths within the employed labour force already outstrip existing training programmes, but they also indicate that few employers are taking any steps to respond effectively, or to prevent further infections (IOM 2004). One reason for this is the high cost of treatment relative to the cost of labour – employers prefer to replace infected workers as they become unable to continue working and provide minimal death and disability benefits to workers and their families, compared with other sectors where employment is more formalised, such as the mining industry. The costs incurred by employers are mainly the product of absenteeism and retraining, and the epidemic's impact on production in the long term has not been estimated. Non-governmental organisations (NGOs) in South Africa and Zimbabwe have reported that HIV-positive farm workers have been evicted when they become too ill to continue working. The epidemic appears to be aggravating longer-term trends in commercial agriculture in South Africa towards casualisation of labour and the forced relocation of (former) farm workers to informal settlements, or in some cases, low-cost housing in nearby towns.

Counter-examples

Existing research describing the devastating and multifaceted impact of HIV/AIDS on affected rural households in communal and commercial farming areas has hypothesised that as the epidemic continues, these same impacts will be magnified. However, this may not happen in a predictable and linear way. In qualitative case study research and in the media, stories are emerging that suggest that the responses of communities to the epidemic are changing, particularly as widows and others affected by HIV/AIDS are starting to organise around livelihood demands. Such outcomes may be atypical, but are nevertheless instructive.

What is evident thus far is that traditional land allocation practices are being increasingly challenged and even, in some places, changed. In KwaZulu-Natal, for example, research has found that chiefs have protected widows from disinheritance by their in-laws and, in the face of mounting demands, have started to allocate land-use rights to single and widowed women and even to child-headed households (IRRD 2002). Contrary to tradition, chiefs and headmen in Lesotho were found to be allowing households affected by HIV/AIDS, and therefore unable to cultivate their land, to retain their rights to the land, even when this was left fallow for several seasons – thereby maintaining their social standing in the community and providing the possibility that they could resume cultivation at a future time (FAO and SARPN 2002). In both instances, researchers have argued that chiefs' concern with the welfare of households in crisis is intermingled with their resistance to attempts by the state to impose new land laws that would erode traditional authority. In this way, some 'compassionate chiefs' have used the epidemic as a means to gain popularity among communities in crisis and to entrench their position, where the institution of customary tenure was under threat. They have done so not only by maintaining custom and tradition, but also by adapting traditional practices of land allocation to a changed environment (FAO and SARPN 2002).

Traditional leaders and local administrators also allocated land to women in the context of Zimbabwe's fast-track land reform and in some instances, rather than being a cause for stigma, HIV status emerged as a basis for affirmative action in allocation of land. Although limited, there were cases where women benefited from fast-track resettlement. In the Seke district near Harare, widows, divorcees and single women have been allocated land under a fast-track resettlement programme. Similar cases are also reported from Chiredzi district. In Seke, the HIV and AIDS support group had lobbied the Seke district administrator to allocate land to people living with HIV and AIDS (PLWHA) and as a result, 5 per cent of land was allocated to PLWHA (Kaori Izumi, e-mail, 2 May 2006. See also Izumi 2006b, 43–44).

Elsewhere, community-based organisations, often comprised of widows and/or women affected by HIV/AIDS, have successfully lobbied for land rights and for support to produce food for themselves and their families – and to raise cash income through collective efforts (for more examples, see Izumi 2006a, 2006b). In Swaziland, Swazis for Positive Living (SWAPOL), organising in more than 30 rural communities, negotiated with chiefs to allocate land to women to cultivate 'nutrition gardens' individually, as well as cropping fields for collective production. They managed to get a woman acting as regent for an under-age chief to lobby other chiefs to allocate land so that they could establish an agricultural co-operative to provide income for the organisation. SWAPOL distributed 25 per cent of profit from the agricultural co-operative to its members, 25 per cent to caring for PLWHA and invested the remaining 50 per cent. In Kenya, Grassroots Organisations Together in Sisterhood (GROOTS) went further by organising input supply and food-purchasing syndicates to enable poor women, mostly widows, to buy cheaply in bulk and to use savings to transport their goods to urban centres, or sell grain to sellers to secure higher returns (IRIN-News 2005; Izumi 2006a). In these instances, women appealed to state and traditional authorities to change established practices, not by challenging tradition, but by pointing to their traditional gendered roles as carers and providers for children as a basis to secure access to land in the context of HIV/AIDS.

Although the examples cited above are anecdotal and may not reflect common trends, they do demonstrate how traditional practices are mutable and open to change when confronted with changing social conditions. The extent to which these new norms take root may well affect the future growth and impact of the epidemic, as well as shaping individual, household and community-level coping strategies. There are also legal and policy changes that could alter current practices and outcomes, including strengthening women and children's property rights by persuading traditional leaders to advocate the allocation of land rights to women; the protection of women and children's inheritance rights; public support for smallholder agricultural production through infrastructure provision, improved extension services and market access for smallholders, as well as provision of public works and non-farm enterprises in rural enterprises as a source of cash income.

These findings are important for other reasons too. The problem with the bulk of the literature on HIV/AIDS and rural livelihoods, and the postulated chain of causality it has embraced, is not only that it is extremely depressing; it is also based on a linear logic and on generalisations that do not, or will not, always hold true. This can lead to agencies being immobilised because the situation seems hopeless. First, the literature has tended to ignore counter-examples, such as those described above. Second, it has drawn attention to rural people only as victims and has ignored the degree to which they have organised collectively around common livelihood struggles in the face of chronic illness and death. It has also downplayed the degree to which, while some households experience deepening crisis as a result of the epidemic, others benefit. Third, current responses to the epidemic are premised on existing trends described in the literature, which are not necessarily a useful predictor of future responses.

In particular, existing impacts and coping strategies have been shaped by the role of older women (and men) in rural areas – the grandmothers onto whom much of the burden of food production and childrearing has passed. But this may not be the case in a generation's time; changes in demography may mean fewer 'granny' headed households in the future, and the burden of care may fall increasingly to a younger generation, or to child-headed households.

Implications for human security and governance

There is, however, an emerging consensus: gender inequality makes the effects of HIV/AIDS on agriculture and on rural livelihoods *worse*. This is because, where women have insecure rights to land, where they have limited opportunities to generate off-farm income and where they have few assets of their own, HIV-affected households are more likely to experience property-grabbing, to lose their land and to be unable to maintain food production (Wiegers and Scott 2004). In view of this reality, policy interventions should strengthen the property and inheritance rights for women and children, particularly their land and housing rights.

A second emerging consensus is that policy interventions should promote low-cost and labour-saving forms of agricultural production. This is an influential perspective promoted by the FAO in developing countries. However, as Scott Drimie and Sithabiso Gandure observe, the FAO's promotion of labour-saving technologies and crops can be criticised for seeking to reduce reliance on the one factor of production that poor people have in relative abundance – their own labour (2005). They argue instead that the impetus towards labour-saving technologies may undermine local labour markets, driving down wages and, in this way, weaken a key income-earning resource of the rural poor.

A third emerging consensus is related to the current and future significance of resource-based conflict and specifically conflict over access to and control of land, particularly in a context of inheritance and contestations over the authority to allocate land. While conflict within and between households, or between households and allocating authorities may be on the rise, it is not clear whether or not this may manifest in broader society-level conflict over land. What is already well documented is the loss of social cohesion in response to the epidemic and what happens to people, particularly OVC, who are separated from family, community and values, over generations. As Catherine Cross, a research specialist at the HSRC, comments: 'If households don't keep the right to land, they don't have the right to exist . . . The sequence goes from Aids to poverty to land snatching to dispossession . . . dropping out of the community is the final risk to Aids survivors.' (cited in SAPA 2003)

Policy implications for rural development

The shift towards mainstreaming HIV/AIDS has barely begun in rural development, agricultural and land policies in southern Africa. If we want to find alternatives in the area of securing rights to land in the region, we need to think through an HIV/AIDS lens. The challenge is to make policy – in all spheres – for an HIV-infected and -affected population: to establish a presumption of an HIV-positive subject.

The mainstreaming of HIV/AIDS in land, agriculture and rural development departments in SADC countries merits further exploration. A study by Esther Wiegers and Melanie Scott found that while the issue had been widely recognised as a personnel matter, few countries in the region had reoriented their agricultural policies to respond to HIV/AIDS in the external service provision environment (2004). In South Africa, for instance, the HIV/AIDS policy of the Department of Land Affairs focuses wholly on HIV in relation to its own employees and does not include the beneficiaries of its land reform programme (2000). Its policies have not explicitly engaged with the question of what kind of land reform is needed for an HIV-infected and -affected population and the implications for a major programme of government, such as land reform, have only started to be explored recently, in a study on the threats of HIV/AIDS to land reform (IFPRI 2006). Despite the focus on HIV/AIDS as a personnel issue, there has been little attention to, and less data collection on, the loss of professionals from the civil service and its implications for service delivery.

To mitigate the impact of HIV/AIDS in the rural areas of southern Africa, a new agenda is needed for agricultural policy. This should promote low-input production, nutritious, non-labour intensive cropping, labour-saving technologies for collecting water and fuel, and investments in livestock as a flexible asset and a source of draught power (VETAID 2003). HIV/AIDS mitigating policies in rural areas would prioritise food production on small plots close to homesteads, allowing women in particular to manage home-based care and basic food production. Priorities for policy advocacy and programming include productivity support, which should focus on interventions with a high food-access-to-input ratio (SADC FANR 2003, v). To enable poor households to generate cash income while minimising risk, states should promote agricultural co-operatives, in which poor smallholders can share the costs of production, as well as marketing, and gain access to agro-processing. Agricultural policies should enable poor people, particularly widows, to access cheap inputs for household food production and support input co-operatives, in order to access these inputs at low cost and in small quantities.

More than ever, we need to move beyond the caricatured notions of full-time farming on economic units of land that continue to prevail in the agricultural establishments and in officialdom through much of the SADC region. These notions were always analytically and pragmatically flawed and have promoted capital-intensive production methods in a context of capital-scarcity. The result in South Africa's land reform programme has been high levels of indebtedness among poor farmers, which has prompted the Land Bank to repossess some farms. In the context of the

HIV/AIDS epidemic, policy emphasis on commercial and full-time farming represents an ideological barrier to finding solutions to the desperate livelihood deficiencies of the rural poor.

It is now widely agreed that a crucial mitigating strategy is the need to change land allocation practices to ensure that women are allocated land in their own right, to support democratic local institutions to administer land rights, maintain records of land rights and adjudicate disputes (Izumi 2006b). This suggests an urgent need for legal reform in the area of marriage and property rights, including customary marriage and the customary laws of inheritance, particularly intestate succession, and legal protection for women's property rights in the context of polygynous marriages.

With regard to HIV/AIDS and property rights in rural areas, there are few examples of best practice, but a few important initiatives do stand out. As part of a programme to strengthen women's property rights, the International Centre for Research on Women (ICRW) supports a small number of initiatives by NGOs in sub-Saharan Africa that examine and address the 'links between HIV/AIDS and the absence of women's and girls' property and inheritance rights' (ICRW 2006, 1). ICRW's programme aims to document these initiatives and to share information about their effectiveness with donor governments, local NGOs and in-country policy-makers. Some of these interventions have driven processes of law reform in marriage, inheritance and land laws in Malawi, Rwanda and Uganda. The initiative is jointly managed by the ICRW, the Global Coalition on Women and AIDS (GCWA) and the FAO, with funds provided by the Joint United Nations Programme on HIV/AIDS (UNAIDS). This initiative is supporting groups such as the Rwanda Women Community Development Network to assist women in a post-conflict and HIV/AIDS-afflicted situation to claim their land rights and to prevent dispossession.

In summary, in rural development, agricultural and land policy, elements of a new policy agenda, which mainstreams HIV/AIDS, include:

- Agricultural policies: to promote low-input land uses, crops, livestock and agricultural technologies that require limited bought seed, fertiliser and pesticides, produce high-quality nutrition and can be cultivated close to the homestead by people involved in home-based care.
- Land allocation practices: to promote equitable allocation of communal land and prioritisation of households living with HIV/AIDS and, in commercial agriculture, to ensure that land is allocated to farm workers for their own use.

- Women's tenure rights: to strengthen the independent tenure rights of women and of children in law and in practice, in both communal areas and on commercial farms.
- Cultural practices: to curb property-grabbing, limit the cost of funeral rites and stop the practice of widows being inherited by their brothers-in-law; to provide greater certainty and gender equality in inheritance and to provide clarity on guardianship and property rights of OVC. (Izumi 2006b)

Conclusions

Despite the burgeoning literature recording the impact of HIV/AIDS in the rural areas and the ways in which it has interacted with and transformed the shape of rural society and livelihoods, there are important gaps in our knowledge. More research is needed to describe and understand the trajectory of this impact and the factors that determine the sequence of phases and the pace at which they proceed. We need to know – and ask – more about factors aggravating or mitigating the impact and about shifting social practices that can change this equation. We need more study of the impact of HIV/AIDS on women and children's property and inheritance rights and on how securing these rights may affect household survival.

There is nevertheless a real danger of reductionist reasoning that proposes that, seen through the lens of HIV/AIDS, all changes and disasters in rural livelihoods are due to the epidemic. Changes and adaptations in livelihood strategies are responses to a set of complex pressures, not only HIV/AIDS. Yet studies of the impact of the epidemic have no control group and thus a multitude of problems and crises may be ascribed to HIV/AIDS, when in fact, these interact with other pressures exerted on rural populations – among them, the dramatic decline in the availability of urban jobs and cash incomes (as in Zimbabwe), declining state support for agricultural production (through much of the region) and drought and fluctuations in weather patterns due to climate change. Those describing and analysing the implications of the epidemic for rural people should bear this in mind.

The durability and adaptability of social institutions, norms and practices will shape the trajectory of the epidemic and its outcomes for rural livelihoods. Because impacts are mediated through social relationships, changes to cultural norms and practices could change the impact of the epidemic over time. Important policy implications flow from this: interventions that advocate change in key social institutions, such as traditional authorities, marriage practices and land tenure could change how rural communities respond to HIV/AIDS and strengthen how they cope with illness and death.

There are also methodological implications. First, there is the danger of aggregation. The literature reported in this chapter has alerted us to dominant trends, but for improvements in policy-making, it is important to understand why people in different situations are differentially affected, or respond differently to a crisis. A priority in future studies is to differentiate the type of impact on households. The impact on poverty is known, but, as Alex de Waal and Joseph Tumushabe argue, it is not clear how differences within the epidemic (the profiles of morbidity and mortality) affect various socio-economic groups within a given society, and what these differences imply about food security (2003). Second is the critical importance of structuring interdisciplinary enquiry and third, there is a need for longitudinal sociological (as opposed to epidemiological) studies to chart the long-term trajectory of individuals, households and communities. These will need to be multi-site, in order to capture variations across countries and across agro-ecological settings.

References

Action Aid. 2006. 'The Johannesburg Position on HIV/AIDS and Women's and Girls' Rights in Africa'. Declaration of the African Women's Regional Consultation on Women's and Girls' Rights and HIV/AIDS in Africa, 6–7 April. Johannesburg.

Baylies, Carolyn. 2002. 'The Impact of Aids on Rural Households in Africa: A Shock like Any Other'. *Development and Change* 33(4): 611–32.

De Waal, Alex and Joseph Tumushabe. 2003. 'HIV/AIDS and Food Security in Africa'. Report for the Department for International Development (DfID), 1 February. United Kingdom.

Department of Land Affairs. 2000. 'HIV/AIDS Policy'. Pretoria: Department of Land Affairs.

Drimie, Scott and Sithabiso Gandure. 2005. *The Impact of HIV/AIDS on Rural Livelihoods in Southern Africa: An Inventory and Literature Review*. Report for the Food and Agricultural Organisation (FAO).

FAO (Food and Agricultural Organisation) and SARPN (Southern African Regional Poverty Network). 2002. 'Report on FAO/SARPN Workshop on HIV/AIDS and Land'. Pretoria, 23–24 June.

FAO News. 2004. 'Protecting Women's Property and Land Rights to Protect Families in AIDS-Affected Communities'. 8 March. Rome: FAO.

FAO-SAFR (Food and Agricultural Organisation – Subregional Office for Southern and East Africa). 2006. *Unite for Children, Unite against AIDS and Property Stripping: Regional Workshop on HIV and AIDS and Children's Property Rights and Livelihoods in Southern and East Africa*. Harare: FAO-SAFR.

Heyzer, Noeleen. 2004. 'Peace of Mind, Piece of Land'. *Our Planet*, special issue, September: Women, Health and the Environment. Available at http://www.ourplanet.com/imgversn/152/heyzer.html, accessed 30 August 2007.

HRC (Human Rights Commission). 2003. 'Inquiry into Human Rights Violations in Farming Communities'. Available at http://www.sahrc.org.za/sahrc_cms/exec/search.cgi, accessed 14 December 2007.

ICRW (International Centre for Research on Women). 2006. 'Reducing Women's and Girls' Vulnerability to HIV/AIDS by Strengthening their Property and Inheritance Rights'. Information newsletter, May.

IFPRI (International Food Policy Research Institute). 2006. 'HIV/AIDS, Land-Based Livelihoods and Land Reform in South Africa'. Report to IFPRI and the Department of Land Affairs, South Africa, January. Compiled by the HSRC, University of Fort Hare, University of KwaZulu-Natal and Nkuzi Development Association.

ILO (International Labour Organisation). 2004. *HIV/AIDS and Work: Global Estimates, Impacts and Response*. Geneva: ILO.

IOM (International Organisation for Migration). 2004. 'Developing Regional Guidelines on HIV and AIDS for the Commercial Agriculture Sector in the SADC Region'. 2–3 December. Centurion.

IRIN-News. 2005. 'Swaziland: HIV-Positive Women's Group Creates Agricultural Cooperative'. 22 February. Available at http://www.irinnews.org/Report.aspx?ReportId=38207, accessed 14 December 2007.

IRRD (Integrated Rural and Regional Development). 2002. *The Impact of HIV/AIDS on Land Issues in KwaZulu-Natal Province, South Africa: Interview Narratives from Muden, Dondotha, Kwadumisa and Kwanyuswa*. June. Pretoria: HSRC.

Izumi, Kaori. 2006a. *Reclaiming Our Lives: HIV and AIDS, Women's Land and Property Rights and Livelihoods in Southern and East Africa: Narratives and Responses*. Pretoria: HSRC, FAO and Global Coalition on Women and AIDS.

———. 2006b. *The Land and Property Rights of Women and Orphans in the Context of HIV and AIDS: Case Studies from Zimbabwe*. Pretoria: HSRC, FAO and Global Coalition on Women and AIDS.

Jayne, Thomas S., Marcela Villareal, Prabhu Pingali and Gunter Hemrich. 2005. 'HIV/AIDS and the Agricultural Sector in Eastern and Southern Africa: Anticipating the Consequences'. Unpublished research paper. Rome: FAO.

Moyo, Sam and Ruth Hall. 2007. 'Conflict and Land Reform in Southern Africa: How Exceptional is South Africa?' In *South Africa in Africa: The Post-Apartheid Decade*, ed. Adekeye Adebajo, Adebayo Adedeji and Chris Landsberg, 150–76. Pietermaritzburg: University of KwaZulu-Natal Press.

Mphale, Matšeliso M., Emmanuel G. Rwambali and Mokhantšo G. Makoae. 2002. *HIV/AIDS and its Impacts on Land Tenure and Livelihoods in Lesotho*. Report for the FAO.

Mutangadura, Gladys B. 2005. 'Gender, HIV and Rural Livelihoods in Southern Africa: Addressing the Challenges'. *Jenda: A Journal of Cultural and African Women Studies* 7: 1–19.

SADC FANR (Southern African Development Community, Food Agriculture and Natural Resources) VAC (Vulnerability Assessment Committee). 2003. *Towards Identifying Impacts of HIV/AIDS on Food Insecurity in Southern Africa and Implications for Response: Findings from Malawi, Zambia and Zimbabwe*. Harare: SADC FANR.

SAMP (Southern African Migration Project). 2004. 'Mainstreaming Migration in Southern Africa'. Briefing for DfID (Department for International Development), August. United Kingdom.

SAPA (South African Press Association). 2003. 'Aids Survivors Risk Dispossession'. *Mail & Guardian* 15 July. Available at http://www.mg.co.za/articledirect.aspx?articleid=24566, accessed 14 December 2007.

Sunde, Jackie and Karin Kleinbooi. 1999. *Promoting Equitable and Sustainable Development for Women Farm Workers in the Western Cape*. Stellenbosch: Centre for Rural Legal Studies.

Tibbo, Karen and Scott Drimie. 2006. 'Chronic Vulnerability and Food Insecurity: An Overview from Southern Africa'. *Humanitarian Exchange* 33, March: 2–4. London: Overseas Development Institute.

Topouzis, Daphne. 1998. 'The Implications of HIV/AIDS for Rural Development Policy and Programming'. UNDP Study Paper 6. New York: UNDP.

VETAID. 2003. *Mitigating the Effects of HIV/AIDS on Food Security and Agriculture in Eastern and Southern Africa*. Summary conference report, 3–7 November. Maputo.

Walker, Lynn. 2002. ' "We Will Bury Ourselves": A Study of Child-Headed Households on Commercial Farms in Zimbabwe'. Harare: Farm Orphan Support Trust of Zimbabwe.

Wiegers, Esther and Melanie Scott. 2004. 'HIV/AIDS, Gender Inequality and the Agricultural Sector: Guidelines for Incorporating HIV/AIDS and Gender Considerations into Agricultural Programming in High Incidence Countries'. Report for Interagency Coalition on AIDS and Development (ICAD), November. Ottawa.

7

Orphans and Security[1]

——— • ———

Robyn Pharoah

Introduction

With an estimated 33 million people living with HIV/AIDS (PLWHA) worldwide, the HIV/AIDS epidemic is now recognised as one of the greatest humanitarian and developmental challenges of our era (UNAIDS 2007, 1). In the hardest-hit regions of the world, the epidemic is increasing poverty and inequality and reversing decades of improvements in health, education and life expectancy. It is also leaving millions of children orphaned and living in situations of acute vulnerability. Yet, even as the international community mobilises in support of these young people, some researchers and practitioners are suggesting that growing numbers of impoverished orphans may pose a threat to individual and communal security in some countries. This chapter explores the evidence for such linkages. It begins by examining the hypothesised implications of the epidemic for security and stability, before going on to examine the state, nature and realities of orphanhood in South Africa and the implications of a more subtle understanding of the security consequences of the epidemic for future policy and programming.

AIDS, orphans and security: The theory

By killing and debilitating large numbers of people, it is widely agreed that AIDS is undermining already fragile families, communities, national economies and governance. It may also be creating or exacerbating social and political disruption and conflict. As Mark Schneider and Michael Moodie argue: 'In much of the developing world, particularly in Africa, AIDS is undermining education and health systems, economic growth, micro-enterprises, policing and military capabilities, political legitimacy, family structures, and overall social cohesion' (2002, 5).

There is an abundance of research on the implications of HIV/AIDS at an individual and household level. Several studies have shown that the wealth and assets of affected households are being reduced and families are being broken up (see, for example, Steinberg et al. 2002; Marcus 1999; Foster and Williamson 2000, 275–84; UNICEF 1999; Foster et al. 1997; Ford and Hosegood 2004). There is also some evidence that in Africa, where over half of the population is already under the age of fifteen, the death of unprecedented numbers of working-age men and women is changing the shape of the population pyramids in heavily affected countries, increasing the proportion of children and youth in these populations (Epstein 2002; UNDESA 2004). The data wear thin at community, national and regional levels, however. Studies indicate that economic productivity may be declining in some heavily affected countries, but there is very little hard evidence available to illuminate the macro-economic, political and stability effects of the epidemic (see CADRE, USAID and the Joint Centre for Political and Economic Studies 2002 for an extensive overview of the available literature). While often presented as fact, much of our current knowledge in this area is based on informed speculation, rather than empirical data. It is argued, however, that by increasing poverty and vulnerability, widening the gap between rich and poor and undermining the credibility and operational effectiveness of states, AIDS may exacerbate or provoke social volatility, political polarisation and conflict.

Within this complex web of multidirectional effects, many analysts are making a link between growing numbers of children orphaned by AIDS and crime or instability. The first and most common argument is that the illness and death of parents will leave children scarred and marginalised in ways that predispose them to delinquency and criminal behaviour. Proponents of this theory believe that growing poverty, together with the emotional trauma associated with multiple AIDS-related deaths and stigma, reduced levels of parental care and the loss of positive role models will place children at high risk of developing antisocial tendencies. Emma Guest, for example, argues:

> Adversity can make people strong, but it will be an unusual AIDS orphan who gains anything from the epidemic. The damage from growing up alone will be deep and, in some cases, permanent . . . child mortality will increase, as will levels of malnutrition, illiteracy and child abuse . . .

the number of children living on the street, fighting wars, committing violent crime, joining gangs and abusing alcohol will rise. (2001, 157)

The second argument is that growing numbers of orphans will provide a recruitment pool for individuals and organisations who want to challenge the existing socio-political order in African countries violently. According to Randy Cheek, a swell of young people without family care and formal schooling may constitute a population group vulnerable to co-option into socially disruptive activities and ethnic warfare (2000, 5). Like many other analysts, he emphasises the threat posed by growing numbers of street children. Describing the implications of the epidemic for society, Cheek says:

> AIDS orphans represent more than just a humanitarian catastrophe. The collapse of traditional support systems, and the resulting proliferation of street orphans, represents a direct threat to regional stability that could result in unprecedented civilian casualties due to ethnic and regional conflict . . . The HIV/AIDS crisis currently ravaging Southern Africa will exact a heavy toll on stability in a region already beset by many critical problems with significant implications for US security planning. (2000, 1)

A third argument is that the demographic change brought about by the epidemic, specifically an overrepresentation of adolescents and young adults in heavily affected populations, will create problems. Martin Schönteich speculates that because young men are most likely to commit crime, a disproportionate number of males between the ages of 15 and 24 in severely affected countries may lead to higher levels of crime – particularly violent crime and group-based aggression (2003, 23). Others argue that by straining social institutions, such as the labour market and educational system, so-called 'youth bulges' resulting from either HIV/AIDS or fertility trends may make countries generally more unstable and prone to violence (see, for example, Cincotta, Engelman and Anastasion 2003, 42–44).

The nature and extent of AIDS-related orphaning in South Africa

The statistics on orphaning vary according to how orphans are defined. Some estimates use data for children under the age of fifteen, while others expand their definitions to include young people under the age of eighteen, with the literature variously reporting on 'maternal orphans' whose mothers have died, 'paternal orphans' whose fathers have died and 'double orphans'.[2] Using an expansive definition of orphanhood (children under the age of eighteen who have lost one or both of their parents), estimates by the Joint United Nations Programme on HIV/AIDS (UNAIDS), United Nations (International) Children's (Emergency) Fund (UNICEF) and the United States Agency for International Development (USAID) suggest that by the end of 2003, 2.2 million South African children – 13 per cent of all children – had lost one or both of their parents. This number is expected to increase to 3.1 million, or 19 per cent of children, by 2010 (2004, 4).

Data from a national study conducted in 2004 by the Nelson Mandela Children's Fund and the Human Sciences Research Council (HSRC) indicate that most orphans had one surviving parent, usually their mother. The findings show that 14.4 per cent of children between the ages of two and eighteen had lost parents, of whom 10 per cent were paternal orphans, 2.6 per cent were maternal orphans and only 2 per cent were double orphans (2005, 112). They also show that the likelihood of being orphaned increases with age, with 21 per cent of children between the ages of fifteen and eighteen reporting being orphaned, compared to 13.3 per cent of two- to fourteen-year-olds. Modelling by Debbie Bradshaw et al. similarly suggests that while 20–30 per cent of ten- to fourteen-year-olds are expected to lose their mothers by 2015, this figure will rise to well over 30 per cent among children between the ages of fifteen and seventeen (cited in Johnson and Dorrington 2001).

It is impossible to say for certain how many children have lost parents to AIDS, but available estimates suggest that the virus is becoming a leading cause of orphaning in South Africa. UNAIDS, UNICEF and USAID estimate that almost half (48 per cent) of all orphans under the age of eighteen have lost parents to the epidemic. The projections by Bradshaw et al. (2002) suggest that a vast majority of children will be orphaned by AIDS by 2015. As shown in Figure 7.1, it is expected that the number of maternal orphans under the age of fifteen orphaned by other causes will gradually decline – as a result of both larger numbers of mothers dying of AIDS and declining levels of fertility – and the number of children orphaned by AIDS will rise enormously over the next decade. The number of children orphaned by AIDS is predicted to peak at about 1.85 million in 2015. If the age limit is extended to include children between the ages of fifteen and eighteen, this figure rises to 3.1 million (Bradshaw et al. 2002, 2).

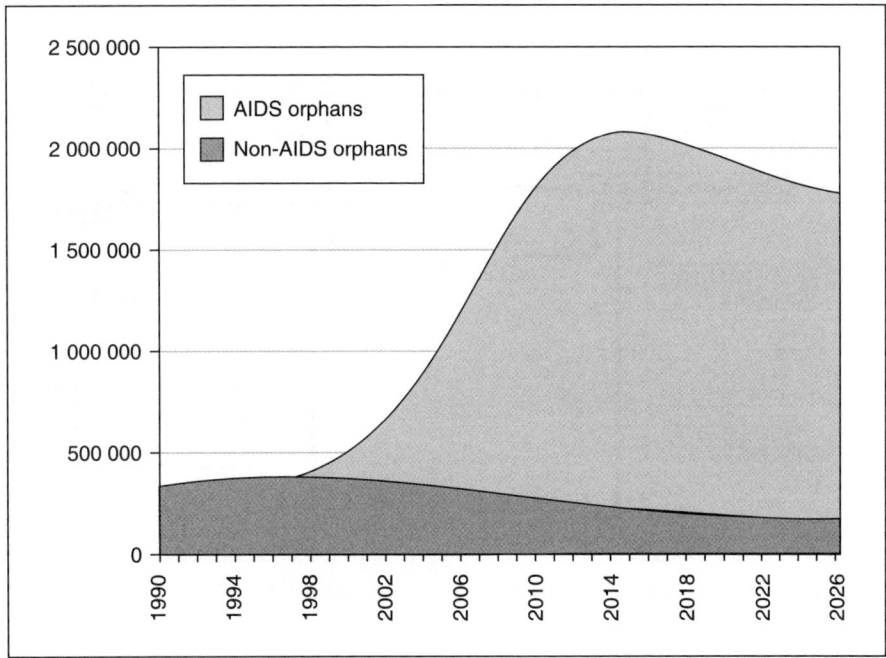

Figure 7.1 The projected number of maternal AIDS and non-AIDS orphans under the age of fifteen by 2015.

Source: Bradshaw et al. 2002

The implications of HIV/AIDS for children

The illness and death of caregivers as a result of AIDS may reduce the well-being of children in several ways. As shown in Figure 7.2, the illness and death of a caregiver may result in children experiencing growing poverty and its correlates: the loss of parental affection, reduced levels of care, stigma and the psycho-social implications of repeated personal and material losses, such as trauma, stress, depression and a loss of friends, family connections and other social relationships. Even before a caregiver's death, children may feel the effects of terminal illness, as they shoulder new responsibilities, such as additional domestic chores, taking care of sick parents, income-generating activities and childcare duties. Research suggests that the educational, social, economic and psychological problems encountered by children may be most severe prior to a parent's death (cited in Foster 2004, 67). Studies show that household income may decline by as much as 40–60 per cent, as breadwinners

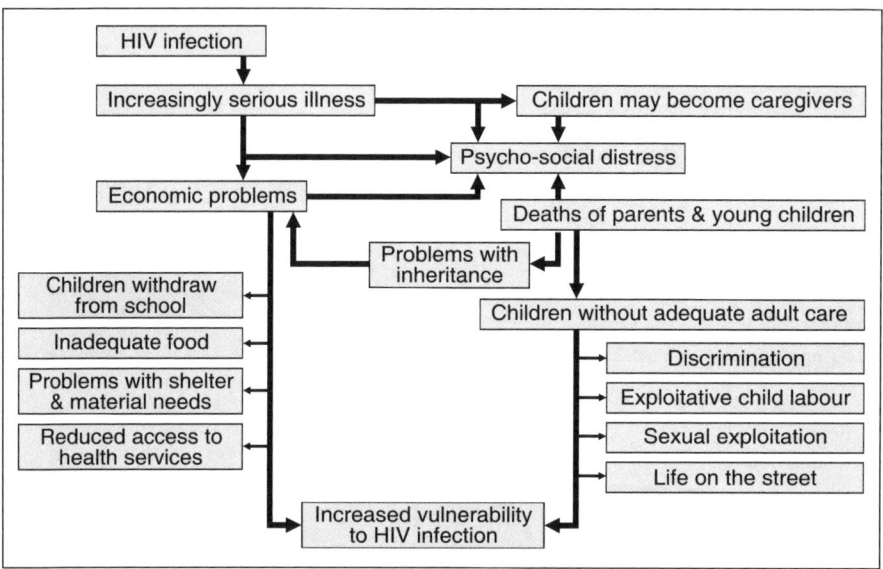

Figure 7.2 Problems among children and families affected by HIV/AIDS.

Source: Williams 2005

become unable to earn and money is spent on healthcare, and later, funeral costs (International Crisis Group 2001, 23; see also Chapters 6 and 10 in this volume). Household asset reserves and savings may also be depleted, as families sell possessions to raise money for healthcare costs and to compensate for a breadwinner's loss of earnings. Children may receive poorer care and supervision at home, suffer from malnutrition and have less access to health services (Richter 2004, 11). Many may be forced to drop out of school, as the money earmarked for school expenses is used for basic necessities and healthcare. Even where there are adequate resources for children to continue their schooling, both the additional duties assumed by affected children and discrimination may cause them to drop out of school (Richter 2004, 12). In some cases, they may also be sent to live with other people, which often results in siblings being separated from one another, further disrupting children's lives and increasing their isolation.[3]

Many of these effects continue after the caregiver's death. Studies in several countries show that income in orphan households may be as much as 20–30 per cent lower than in non-orphaned households (Foster and Williamson 2000). Some comparative studies on how children orphaned by AIDS fare compared with non-orphans in a range of African settings show that orphans suffer higher levels of malnutrition than non-orphans (see, for example, Stein 2003, 7) and are less likely to attend school (UNICEF cited in Richter 2004, 10; Foster and Williamson 2000). Participatory research shows that children often face discrimination within their families, communities, churches and schools (see, for example, Save the Children 2001, 15–25; Tolfree 2004, 65). There is also anecdotal evidence that orphans may experience high levels of economic and sexual abuse, although there do not appear to be any studies examining the prevalence of abuse compared to other children (Foster 2004, 68). Death and migration may also result in the creation of child-headed households, or in children living on the street. Due to the conditions of mutual dependency that often exist between adult and child orphans who go to live with relatives, live in child-headed households, or are left to fend for themselves, youngsters may find themselves in precarious circumstances, especially where they are cared for by elderly relatives (Richter 2004, 10).

Deepening poverty and the multiple losses associated with AIDS-related illness and death, stigma, discrimination and migration – including the loss of family members, siblings, friends, familiar surroundings, schooling opportunities and, in many ways, childhood – may result in considerable psycho-social stress. There are only a handful of studies on the implications of AIDS-related illness and death for the psychological, emotional and social adjustment of children. Research in KwaZulu-Natal, for example, found that youngsters whose parents had AIDS were often extremely anxious about their illness, to the point that they had difficulty concentrating at school (Marcus 1999, 22). Five other African studies, which compared orphans to non-orphans from the same community, suggest that orphans not only experience more anxiety, but also more depression than other children. None of the studies, however, showed that orphaned children are any more prone to delinquency, with the available evidence suggesting that orphans tend to show internalising behaviour, such as depression, anxiety and withdrawal, rather than aggression and other forms of antisocial behaviour (see Stein 2003, 9–10 for a review of available studies).

Many studies also show that that not all children are equally vulnerable and that children orphaned by AIDS are often no more disadvantaged than poor children living in comparable circumstances. This suggests that the implications of orphanhood vary according to context and that the boundaries between children orphaned by AIDS and other orphans and vulnerable children are frequently blurred.

AIDS orphaning in context

Donald Skinner et al. argue that many commentaries on the situation of children affected by HIV/AIDS, and orphans in particular, tend to sensationalise the issue, with the most serious and abhorrent cases identified and extrapolated to describe all orphans in a particular area or region (2004, 2). The picture painted often conjures up images of hordes of traumatised, unwanted children being cast to the very outer fringes of society and left to fend for themselves in a world where life is often 'short, harsh and cheap', but the reality is more complex.

As South African data show, only a relatively small proportion of children are double orphans and children most often have a surviving parent, usually their mother. It is difficult to obtain accurate estimates of the numbers of children living in extremely vulnerable situations, but several African studies suggest that less than 2–3 per cent of orphans live in environments where they are completely without support or where they are exploited (Foster 2004, 70). The Nelson Mandela Children's Fund/HSRC study found that only 3 per cent of the children surveyed were living in households headed by someone under the age of eighteen (2005, 113). A census of children living in two communities in the Free State and North West province carried out by the HSRC in 2003 and 2004 similarly found that only 63 of the 17 950 households surveyed (0.3 percent) were headed by children (Jooste, Managa and Simbayi 2006, 13 and 21). These low numbers suggest that while increasing numbers of orphans may be straining traditional coping mechanisms, such as the extended family, they are still remarkably intact and surprisingly small numbers of children have so far found themselves without the support they have historically provided.

The available data also suggest that even in the absence of HIV/AIDS, many children are not raised in the ideal, stable family environments that much of the literature takes as its starting point. Numerous studies show that large numbers of children in southern Africa have 'lost' parents through the physical and social movements associated with migrant labour and fluid marital and partnership arrangements (Bray 2003, 9). Even where parents are alive, fostering, or the care of non-biological children whose parents live elsewhere, is common. For example, data from the South African Project for Statistics on Living Standards and Development survey (SALSS) conducted in 1993 show that roughly 17 per cent of African children between the ages of six and nineteen were living apart from their biological parents, while 12 per cent of coloured and just under 5 per cent of Indian and white children were fostered (Richter 2004, 18).

The implications of AIDS-related illness and death are also seldom confined to households who lose members to the epidemic. Geoff Foster argues that children not immediately touched by the virus may feel the effects of HIV/AIDS when families provide money to support sick relatives, their mothers leave home to provide care, or their standard of living deteriorates as their family takes in orphaned children (2004, 67). As the epidemic takes hold, they may also be affected as government services and structures tasked with providing for vulnerable children become overstretched (Foster and Williamson 2000 cited in Stein 2003, 5) and as economies affected by the epidemic provide fewer jobs. High levels of illness and death may also have an insidious psycho-social impact. Beverley Killian notes that South African children living in severely affected areas are excessively anxious about death and often reflect obsessively about illness and mortality (2004, 40).

Such dynamics, together with the high levels of poverty that exist in many of the communities worst affected by the epidemic, mean that few of the above problems are confined to children who lose parents to AIDS. As Mamphela Ramphele notes, the loss and absence of parents, insecurity and emotional trauma characterise the lives of many poor children in South Africa:

> Whereas the family is supposed to create a safe haven in life's troubled waters . . . uncertainty permeates family life in a manner that is difficult for outsiders to comprehend. The family unit cannot be taken for granted and the availability of a mother, let alone both parents, is a luxury few children enjoy . . . the provision of basic needs is beyond many, and trusting and respectful relationships are an exception rather than the rule. (2002, 154)

The experience of practitioners, caregivers and children supports this view. Research by the HSRC among service providers, orphans, caretakers of orphans and other stakeholders in eleven communities in Zimbabwe, Botswana and South Africa shows that respondents to surveys associated vulnerability with a range of factors, such as a lack of financial resources, a lack of care and love, overcrowded living conditions, high levels of poverty and exposure to unsafe environments that may or may not be associated with orphanhood. Respondents were at pains to point out that not all children exposed to risks are equally vulnerable. They argued that levels of vulnerability vary over time and may be mediated by the age at which children lose their parents, as well as the assets and internal resources of the child. Respondents identified children with no caregivers, especially street children, as the most vulnerable. Orphans without guardians were deemed more vulnerable than those who had someone to take care of them, with respondents noting that not all orphans are vulnerable and that vulnerability is linked to the quality of care, rather than a particular status (Skinner et al. 2004, 9–13).

An overlap in experience between children orphaned by AIDS and other children necessitates a shift in perspective. The available evidence suggests that although children orphaned by AIDS are affected negatively by their parents' deaths, there is little about these children that should make them disproportionately more likely to turn to crime and violence than other poor children. Rather than focusing on whether children orphaned by the epidemic pose a peculiar threat to stability and security, we should look at how HIV/AIDS may create an environment in which the deepening poverty and vulnerability of a larger group of children, together with demographic change, encourages greater levels of criminality and social and political volatility.

Linkages between AIDS and crime

Pinpointing the causes of crime is a slippery and difficult undertaking, but a broad reading of criminological literature suggests that demographic change, growing levels of poverty and inequality and compromised service delivery may be associated with higher levels of crime and violence – although as yet, there is little evidence of such effects. Factors such as material need, inequity, social exclusion, unemployment, poor education and family breakdown, for example, lie at the heart of many of the prevailing theories of why individuals commit crimes. Factors such as urbanisation and its correlates – which could be exacerbated by the growing economic hardship associated with the epidemic – have also been linked to higher levels of criminality all over the world.

At the micro-level, there are a number of relevant personal, family and environmental variables. As noted by Schönteich, biographical factors, such as age and gender, are closely correlated with criminality, with official arrest and victimisation figures from around the world showing that most crime is committed by young men (Maree 2003, 68). The relationship between crime and age is particularly strong. As David Smith notes, 'probably the most important single fact about crime is that it is committed mainly by teenagers and young adults' (1995,

395). Data from the United States for the years 1980, 1994 and 2000, for example, show that arrest rates for both violent and property crimes increased dramatically among adolescents in their early teens, peaked around the age of eighteen and then decreased continually after the age of twenty (Ezel and Cohen 2005, 1–2).

There is also a range of purely social variables associated with a greater propensity towards criminal behaviour. These include family variables, such as growing up in a single-parent family; poor levels of supervision; having family members who are involved in criminal behaviour and exposure to strife, violence and abuse. They also include schooling variables, such as a lack of formal education, failing or dropping out of school, as well as exposure to overcrowded and unsupportive school environments (see, for example, Booysens 2003; Maree 2003, 55–59; Centre for Research on Youth at Risk 2002; Goldblatt 1998, 123).

The literature also shows that crime is a complex phenomenon and while the factors shown in Table 7.1 clearly influence criminality, the relationships are neither simple nor linear. For instance, although poverty is often a motivating factor, it is not true that the poorest societies have the highest rates of crime, or that the poorest people necessarily commit the most crime (see, for example, Leggett 2002, 3). Similarly, although inequality is more consistently correlated with crime than poverty,

Table 7.1 Risk factors for criminal behaviour.

Broad area	Specific risk factors
Individual	An economically stressed family, violence and physical abuse, sexual abuse, poor parental monitoring and support, loveless parents, lack of supervision, parents using alcohol and/or drugs and negative relationships with parents
Family or home factors	Feeling that life is oppressive, lacking hope for the future, feeling alienated, difficult personality, brain disease disorder, early aggressive behaviour and exposure to different forms of criminal activity
School factors	Lack of education, poor academic performance, failing, truancy, problems at school and poor schooling
Community factors	Poverty, neighbourhood with a high crime rate and unemployment
Extra-family relationships	Associations with deviant peers and gangs

Source: Maree 2003

economic disparities are not always associated with high levels of victimisation. Some of the most unequal societies in the world, such as several of the Arab states, have very low levels of crime (Leggett 2002, 4).

A growing literature on risk and resilience also shows that even where levels of offending are high, the decision to engage in crime remains an individual choice (Leggett 2002, 1) and exposure to micro-level risk factors does not necessarily condemn a child to problems in later life (Maree 2003, 73; Centre for Research on Youth at Risk 2002, 2). Work by James Garbarino and others in the United States shows that the impact of risk factors is highly dependent on children's surroundings, and it is only when three or more risk factors combine with an overwhelming and unsupportive environment that children are likely to become delinquent or violent (cited in Roper 2002, 70). The likelihood of long-term maladjustment is therefore dependent on the form, number and severity of precipitating stresses, as well as the availability of conditions for recovery (Richter 2004, 23). Even low levels of support in childhood appear to enable some children to overcome severe disadvantages (Karsten Hundeide cited in Richter 2004, 22) and it is estimated that less than one-third of children raised in situations of poverty and deprivation are affected negatively by these experiences (Richter 2004, 22).

Crime is also linked to both the opportunities for committing offences and the cost and likelihood of being caught. Even where poverty and vulnerability are high, the likelihood of individuals breaking the law is mediated by factors such as social norms concerning the acceptability of crime, the availability of firearms and other weapons, and the strength of a country's criminal justice institutions. Countries with weak gun or border controls and ineffective criminal justice systems, for example, are likely to experience higher levels of crime than those in which guns are harder to obtain and criminals stand a greater chance of being caught and punished (see, for example, Weiss 2004, 107). Violent crime may also be, at least in part, linked to attitudes to violence. How the HIV/AIDS epidemic impacts on crime will thus be intricately connected to how the effects of the epidemic play themselves out in particular settings, the prevailing macro-economic and social environment, as well as structural factors, such as the availability and acceptability of firearms or other weaponry.

The linkages between the HIV/AIDS epidemic and instability

There is less empirical support for the possible linkages between the epidemic and social and political volatility. A small number of studies have found a relationship between disproportionately high numbers of male youth and the likelihood of both civil war and coalitional aggression – or violence perpetrated by groups, rather than individuals – but there is no proven causality (see, for example, Urdal 2004, 16; Cincotta, Engelman and Anastasion 2003, 40–49). As Joao Porto notes, there is no single cause of a conflict. Among the most commonly cited correlates are competition for environmental and economic resources and markets, political ideology, ethnic and historical rivalries, and a desire for self-determination, dominance, equality and revenge. However, it is the combination and recombination of such factors that result in conflict, rather than their presence per se (FEWER 2001, 7). The available evidence suggests that political instability requires more than simply large numbers of youth in a population and that demographic processes 'do not act alone in producing stresses that can challenge government leadership and the functional capacity of states' (Cincotta, Engelman and Anastasion 2003, 12). As noted by Nicolas Argenti:

> Youth are often cynically mobilised by political leaderships in pursuit of taking and retaining power. But what the overriding majority of the analyses available to us suggest is that young people do not turn to crime or violence *ex nihilo* by some obscure magnetism, but in response to particular historical, economic, and political conditions . . . Violence is not an end in itself for young people any more than it is for anybody else, but a means to an end learned by young people from their elders and used by them when denied all other means. (De Waal and Argenti 2002, 150)

When young rebels in Sierra Leone embarked on a campaign of amputation during the country's eleven-year war, for instance, there were multiple factors at work. One such factor was the youth demographic, but equally important was an environment that made the large-scale co-option of youth into armed groups possible. The components of this environment included politics (a patrimonial system in which many adolescents felt stifled and excluded), poverty and displacement, with war specifically targeting institutions of safety for young people, such as schools and families (Richards 1996, 28). Rebel leaders methodically broke down new recruits' resistance to violence by forcing them to murder their parents and family members, rape other young people and burn their own villages (these abuses are well documented; see, for example, Richards 1996). Such elements were specific to the political, economic and social history of the war in Sierra Leone and it is highly unlikely that they would be replicated in a different context.

Growing levels of AIDS-induced poverty and inequality and poorer macro-economic performance may contribute to generally higher levels of political and social volatility. Ultimately, however, each conflict has a different instability equation or set of equations and it is impossible to predict the likelihood of such outcomes. As Jenny Clover argues, vulnerability is generated and cannot be decontextualised. No situation is universal and each country presents a specific and unique set of interacting factors that oscillate and concatenate over time, to both generate and reduce vulnerability (2003, 6).

Where to from here?

These findings suggest that while there is likely to be a relationship between the dynamics triggered by the HIV/AIDS epidemic and security, and crime in particular, it is difficult to predict the magnitude of these effects. There is currently too little information available on the links between HIV/AIDS and crime and instability to draw definitive conclusions about possible linkages. The evidence that we do have suggests that given appropriate support and viable opportunities for economic and social inclusion, children are unlikely to turn to either crime or violence. Simply labelling children as a threat to security is thus not only overly simplistic, but also risks increasing the stigma and discrimination to which children orphaned by AIDS are already exposed, and may exacerbate, rather than ameliorate, security concerns.

It is beyond dispute that millions of children will lose parents in the decades to come and that these children will suffer the economic, physical and psycho-social implications of both the prolonged illness of their caregivers and their deaths. While it is open to question whether these impacts will play out in a way that threatens the personal safety of large numbers of people, or the existing socio-political order, the epidemic poses an unprecedented challenge to the well-being of families and children in South Africa. It is vital, given the extent of both the human suffering heralded by the epidemic and the possible effects of the epidemic on more traditional security concerns, that mechanisms be put in place to support children and the families and communities that provide the cornerstones for their protection.

There is a vast literature dedicated to elucidating possible support strategies and a thorough discussion of the available policy options is beyond the scope of this chapter. However, several broad approaches to mitigating the effects of the epidemic on children and families can be identified. The most important of these is the move away from a focus on children orphaned by AIDS, or even orphans, to approaches that address the background poverty affecting a larger group of vulnerable children, only some of whom may be orphaned. The second entails supporting not only children's physical and material needs, but also their emotional and social needs. While the magnitude and urgency of the responses required have, until recently, encouraged a reactive approach that prioritises the basic needs of youngsters to healthcare, nutrition, shelter, clothing and education, children have other key developmental requirements, such as the need for secure attachments to significant others and opportunities for self-actualisation (Wilson et al. 2002, 14). This requires strategies that incorporate physical, emotional, mental and spiritual dimensions (Germann 2004, 97). The third shift evident in the literature is a move away from institutionalised care to the provision of support for family or community-based care.

In this context, UNAIDS, UNICEF and USAID suggest a set of principles and strategies for use in programming for orphans and vulnerable children. These principles are guided by both global human rights and the *Convention on the Rights of the Child* (OHCHR 1989) and provide a normative framework for action in support of children affected by HIV and AIDS. They suggest that strategies should aim to:

- strengthen the protection and care of orphans and vulnerable children within their extended families and communities;
- strengthen the economic coping capacity of families and communities;
- enhance the capacity of families and communities to respond to the psycho-social needs and rights of orphans and other vulnerable children, as well as their caregivers;
- link HIV/AIDS prevention activities and care and support for PLWHA to efforts to support orphans and other vulnerable children;
- focus on the most vulnerable children and communities, not only those orphaned by AIDS;
- give particular attention to gender- and age-related roles and address gender discrimination;
- ensure the full involvement of young people;
- strengthen schools and ensure access to education;
- reduce stigma and discrimination;

- accelerate learning and information exchange;
- strengthen partners and partnerships at all levels and build coalitions among key stakeholders; and
- ensure that external support strengthens and does not undermine community initiative and motivation. (UNAIDS, UNICEF and USAID cited in Germann 2004)

In emphasising holistic support of children, these principles represent a shift from a needs-based to a rights-based model of support, which focuses on the whole child and promotes the effective realisation of all their rights. In terms of this model, programmes are challenged to move from a service delivery mode to an advocacy and community mobilisation approach that helps to fulfil the rights of all vulnerable children (UNAIDS, UNICEF and USAID cited in Germann 2004). There is considerable debate, both internationally and in South Africa, about what strategies will best translate such principles into practice. However, agreeing with several other commentators (for example, UNAIDS, UNICEF and USAID), Bradshaw et al. (2002) suggest several reinforcing strategies that South Africa could pursue in order to address the long-term consequences of the epidemic:

- Strengthening of community-based care: community mechanisms to support the care of orphans should be strengthened. Structures and mechanisms should also be established to identify and safeguard the rights of both orphaned and vulnerable children, by better protecting youngsters against abuse and assisting children and families to obtain child welfare grants and access healthcare and education services.
- Exploring innovative care options: creative community-based care approaches should be tested and applied. There is a range of possible options, including placing caregivers in the homes of orphaned children and identifying and hiring surrogate mothers to look after several orphans in homes within communities. Such approaches have been pioneered by groups such as the Durban Child Welfare Society. Their community family care model provides a family-type arrangement for up to six children in their communities of origin, or a similar social context. The community selects, assesses and trains an appropriate community member who becomes a full-time 'mother' to a group of children. Sibling groups are accommodated and new 'families' are created for children who have no contactable relatives (Foster 2004, 84).

- Creating an enabling environment: all forms of state support should be expanded. The Child Care Act should be modified to allow alternative placement options for children in need of care and support, while the care dependency grant should be extended to cater for caregivers looking after children with HIV/AIDS. A general widening of the social security safety net would help to support children within informal systems of care and could be brought about by extending the child support grant to all children below the age of eighteen and removing the means test currently governing the provision of this grant.
- Promoting community-based systems of orphan support: government initiatives with regard to home-based care should be extended to include children. The provision of home-based care and psycho-social support by non-governmental and community-based organisations should also be promoted and strengthened.
- Making antiretroviral (ARV) treatment freely available: little can be done to reduce the number of orphaned children without a comprehensive, accessible national ARV treatment programme. Efforts must be made by all parties to support and hasten the roll-out of treatment to all HIV-positive adults and children.

Helen Meintjies et al. argue that while resources should be aimed at helping families and communities support orphaned and vulnerable children, the foster care system should also be protected and strengthened to better accommodate those children who still require the state to intervene in their care arrangements. More generally, such strategies need to be matched with effective monitoring mechanisms, as well as efforts to improve the accessibility and responsiveness of the current social support system (2003, 54). Access to social support grants, for instance, is hampered by difficulties in obtaining documentation, such as birth and identity records and existing processes need to be improved significantly, if the system is to be either strengthened or expanded. Interventions also need to be sensitive to the realities of orphaning in South Africa. The bulk of polices and programmes aimed at supporting orphaned and vulnerable children focus on very young children, with relatively few targeting adolescent children. Given the higher levels of orphaning among youngsters in their mid-to-late teens, it is vital that programmes include children in this age group.

Implementing such principles will be an enormous undertaking that will require not only significant financial investments on the part of governmental, non-governmental and international organisations, but also political will, capacity-building and the rethinking and reworking of traditional approaches to child welfare and care. Social support mechanisms will need to be reinforced through broader improvements in healthcare and education and the mainstreaming of both HIV/AIDS and support issues into service delivery. No single government department can take responsibility for supporting orphaned and vulnerable children, and effective policy responses will also require a multi-sectoral and interdisciplinary approach.

The makings of more holistic strategies to address the needs of children affected by HIV/AIDS are already in place. Non-governmental actors are increasingly implementing strategies to comprehensively address the needs of vulnerable children. The government's 'National Action Plan for Orphans and Other Children Made Vulnerable by HIV/AIDS, 2006–28' also establishes a basis for the protection and provision of broad-based and integrated developmental services for children affected by the epidemic. The plan advocates expanded treatment for infected children and their families, psycho-social support, the development and strengthening of community-based care models, the creation of a supportive policy and administrative environment, and the mainstreaming of children's issues throughout the public service (DoH 2005). The successful implementation of this framework will require confronting problems such as the generally fragmented nature of governmental service delivery in South Africa and the difficulties of driving and implementing multi-sectoral initiatives in the face of human and financial constraints. Effective action will also have to address the challenges of scaling up promising local activities. There are no simple remedies for such blockages and mobilising the necessary will and resources will be difficult, but necessary. A failure to spend and respond vigorously in the short term will result in an escalation of the long-term costs to society (Bradshaw et al. 2002, 4).

Conclusion

The HIV/AIDS epidemic will cause major social changes in South Africa and will change the face of communities and societies in ways that are still hard to comprehend. The epidemic poses a significant humanitarian challenge. In the absence of appropriate support mechanisms, the growing levels of poverty and vulnerability could also encourage higher levels of crime and violence, although the magnitude of these effects is difficult to predict. Families and local communities have to date demonstrated remarkable resilience and creativity in addressing the myriad needs of affected children and surprisingly few have been left in situations of extreme vulnerability. This resilience must be built and strengthened and decisive action needs to be taken by stakeholders at all levels to mobilise the human and financial resources necessary to successfully implement comprehensive support mechanisms for orphaned and vulnerable children in South Africa.

Notes

1. This chapter draws heavily on Pharoah and Weiss (2005). My thanks to Taya Weiss for her analysis on youth and conflict in West Africa.
2. Some definitions also consider children whose mother is seriously, terminally ill as maternal orphans, as the inability of mothers to provide care in these situations results in children becoming de facto orphans, despite their parents being alive.
3. According to Hunter and Williamson (2000), 'orphaned children' refers to children who have lost either their mother or both their parents, or whose mother is terminally ill.

References

Booysens, Karen. 2003. 'The Relative Nature and Extent of Child and Youth Misbehaviour in South Africa'. In Child and Youth Misbehaviour in South Africa: A Holistic View, ed. Christiaan Bezuidenhout and Sandra Joubert. Pretoria: Van Schaik.

Bradshaw, Debbie, Leigh Johnson, Helen Schneider, David Bourne and Rob Dorrington. 2002. 'Orphans of the HIV/AIDS Epidemic: The Time to Act is Now'. MRC Policy Brief 2, Medical Research Council.

Bray, Rachel. 2003. 'Predicting the Social Consequences of Orphanhood in South Africa'. CSSR Working Paper 29, February. University of Cape Town: Centre for Social Science Research.

CADRE (Centre for AIDS Research), USAID (United States Agency for International Development) and the Joint Centre for Political and Economic Studies. 2002. 'HIV/AIDS, Economics and Governance in South Africa: Key Issues in Understanding Response'. Report, July.

Centre for Research on Youth at Risk. 2002. 'Youth Risk Factors'. Available at http://www.stthomasu.ca/research/youth/risk.htm, accessed 2 March 2005.

Cheek, Randy. 2000. 'A Generation at Risk: Security Implications of the HIV/AIDS Crisis in Southern Africa'. Paper prepared for the National Defence University, Institute for National Strategic Studies, Washington, DC.

Cincotta, Richard, Robert Engelman and Daneile Anastasion. 2003. 'The Security Demographic: Population and Civil Conflict after the Cold War'. Report published by Population Action International, Washington, DC.

Clover, Jenny. 2003. 'UNAIDS Project AIDS in Africa: Scenarios for the Future Conflict as a Stressor in Africa'. Unpublished report prepared by the ISS African Security Analysis Programme for UNAIDS in Africa, Scenarios for the Future Project.

De Waal, Alex and Nicolas Argenti (eds.). 2002. *Young Africa: Realising the Rights of Children and Youth.* Trenton: Africa World Press.

DoH (Department of Health). 2005. 'National Action Plan for Orphans and Other Children Made Vulnerable by HIV/AIDS, 2006-28'. Pretoria: DoH.

Epstein, B. 2002. 'The Demographic Impact of AIDS'. Unpublished report by the US Census Bureau.

Ezel, Michael and Lawrence Cohen. 2005. *Desisting from Crime: Continuity and Change in Long-Term Crime Patterns of Serious Chronic Offenders.* Clarendon Studies in Criminology. Oxford: Oxford University Press.

Ford, Kathleen and Victoria Hosegood. 2004. 'AIDS Mortality and the Mobility of Children in KwaZulu-Natal, South Africa'. Paper presented at the 2004 meeting of the Population Association of America, Boston, 1-3 April.

FEWER (Forum on Early Warning and Early Response). 2001. *Conflict Analysis and Response Definition.* London, April.

Foster, Geoff. 2004. 'Safety Nets for Children Affected by HIV/AIDS in Southern Africa'. In *A Generation at Risk? HIV/AIDS, Vulnerable Children and Security in Southern Africa,* ed. Robyn Pharoah. Institute for Security Studies Monograph Series 109, December.

Foster, Geoff, Choice Makufa, Roger Drew and Etta Kralovec. 1997. 'Factors Leading to the Establishment of Child-Headed Households: The Case of Zimbabwe'. *Health Transition Review* 7: 155-68.

Foster, Geoff and John Williamson. 2000. 'A Review of Current Literature of the Impact of HIV/ AIDS on Children in Sub-Saharan Africa'. *AIDS* 14, supplement 3.

Germann, Stefan. 2004. 'Call to Action: What Do We Do?' In *A Generation at Risk? HIV/AIDS, Vulnerable Children and Security in Southern Africa,* ed. Robyn Pharoah. Institute for Security Studies Monograph Series 109, December.

Goldblatt, Peter. 1998. 'Comparative Effectiveness of Different Approaches'. In *Reducing Offending: An Assessment of Research Evidence on Ways of Dealing with Offending Behaviour,* ed. Peter Goldblatt and Chris Lewis. Home Office Research Studies 187.

Guest, Emma. 2001. *Children of AIDS: Africa's Orphan Crisis.* London and Sterling, Virginia: Pluto; Pietermaritzburg: University of Natal Press.

Hunter, Susan and John Williamson. 2000. 'Children on the Brink'. Report. Washington, DC: USAID.

International Crisis Group. 2001. 'HIV/AIDS as a Security Issue'. Report. Washington, DC.

Johnson, Leigh and Rob Dorrington. 2001. *The Impact of AIDS on Orphanhood in South Africa: A Quantitative Analysis.* Cape Town: Centre for Actuarial Research, University of Cape Town, Monograph 49. Available at http://www.commerce.uct.ac.za/care, accessed 10 April 2006.

Jooste, Sean, Azwifeneli Managa and Leickness Simbayi. 2006. *A Census Report of Orphaned and*

Vulnerable Children in Two South African Communities. Cape Town: Social Aspects of HIV/AIDS and Health Research Programme, HSRC.

Killian, Beverley. 2004. 'Risk and Resilience'. In *A Generation at Risk? HIV/AIDS, Vulnerable Children and Security in Southern Africa*, ed. Robyn Pharoah. Institute for Security Studies Monograph Series 109, December.

Leggett, Ted. 2002. 'The Relationship between Poverty, Inequality and Crime in South Africa'. Unpublished paper prepared for the Office of the South African Presidency, November.

Marcus, Tessa. 1999. 'Living and Dying with AIDS'. Unpublished report prepared for the Children in Distress Network (CINDI), Pietermaritzburg, July.

Maree, Alice. 2003. 'Criminogenic Risk Factors for Youth Offenders'. In *Child and Youth Misbehaviour in South Africa: A Holistic View*, ed. Christiaan Bezuidenhout and Sandra Joubert. Pretoria: Van Schaik.

Meintjies, Helen, Debbie Budlender, Sonja Giese and Leigh Johnson. 2003. 'Children "in Need of Care" or in Need of Cash?' Joint working paper by the Children's Institute and the Centre for Actuarial Research, University of Cape Town, December.

Nelson Mandela Children's Fund/HSRC (Human Sciences Research Council). 2005. *South African National HIV Prevalence, HIV Incidence, Behaviour and Communication Survey, 2005*. Pretoria: HSRC Press.

OHCHR (Office of the High Commissioner for Human Rights). 1989. *Convention on the Rights of the Child*. 20 November. New York: United Nations.

Pharoah, Robyn (ed.). 2004. *A Generation at Risk? HIV/AIDS, Vulnerable Children and Security in Southern Africa*. Institute for Security Studies Monograph Series 109, December.

Pharoah, Robyn and Martin Schönteich. 2003. 'AIDS, Security and Governance in Southern Africa: Exploring the Impact'. ISS Paper 65, January. Institute for Security Studies.

Pharoah, Robyn and Taya Weiss. 2005. 'AIDS, Orphans, Crime and Instability: Exploring the Linkages'. Paper written for the Institute for Security Studies.

Ramphele, Mamphela. 2002. *Steering by the Stars: Being Young in South Africa*. Cape Town: Tafelberg.

Richards, Paul. 1996. *Fighting for the Rain Forest: War, Youth, and Resources in Sierra Leone*. London: James Currey.

Richter, Linda. 2004. 'The Impact of HIV/AIDS on the Development of Children'. In *A Generation at Risk? HIV/AIDS, Vulnerable Children and Security in Southern Africa*, ed. Robyn Pharoah. Institute for Security Studies Monograph Series 109, December.

Roper, Margaret. 2002. 'Kids First: Approaching School Safety'. In *Crime Prevention Partnerships: Lessons from Practice*, ed. Eric Pelser. Pretoria: Institute for Security Studies.

Save the Children. 2001. 'The Role of Stigma and Discrimination in Increasing the Vulnerability of Children and Youth Infected with and Affected by HIV/AIDS'. Report published by Save the Children, South Africa.

Schneider, Mark and Michael Moodie. 2002. *The Destabilising Impacts of HIV/AIDS*. New York: Centre for Strategic and International Studies (CSIS) HIV/AIDS Task Force.

Schönteich, Martin. 1999. 'AIDS and Age: SA's Crime Time Bomb'. *AIDS Analysis Africa* 10(2): 1–2.

———. 2003. 'HIV/AIDS, Policing and Crime in South Africa: Exploring the Impact'. Draft working paper for the CSIS Task Force on HIV/AIDS, February.

Skinner, D., N. Tsheko, S. Mtero-Munati, M. Segwabe, P. Chibatamoto, S. Mfecane, B. Chandiwana, N. Nkomo, S. Tlou and G. Chitiyo. 2004. 'Defining Orphaned and Vulnerable Children'. Social Aspects of HIV/AIDS and Health Research Programme, Occasional Paper 2. Pretoria: HSRC.

Smith, David. 1995. 'Youth Crime and Conduct Disorders'. In *Psychological Disorders in Young People: Time Trends and Their Correlates*, ed. Michael Rutter and David Smith. Chichester: Wiley.

Stein, Jo. 2003. 'Sorrow Makes Children of Us All: A Literature Review on the Psychosocial Impact of HIV/AIDS on Children'. CSSR Working Paper 47. Cape Town: University of Cape Town, Centre for Social Science Research.

Steinberg, Malcolm, Saul Johnson, Gill Schierhout and David Ndegwa. 2002. 'Hitting Home: How Households Cope with the Impacts of the HIV/AIDS Epidemic'. Report published by the Henry J. Kaiser Foundation, Washington, DC.

Tolfree, David. 2004. *Whose Children: Separated Children's Protection and Participation in Emergencies*. Sweden: Save the Children.

UNAIDS (Joint United Nations Programme on HIV/AIDS). 2007. 'AIDS Epidemic Update'. New York and Geneva: United Nations.

UNAIDS (Joint United Nations Programme on HIV/AIDS), UNICEF (United Nations (International) Children's (Emergency) Fund) and USAID (United States Agency for International Development). 2004. *Children on the Brink 2004: A Joint Report of New Orphan Estimates and a Framework for Action*. Washington, DC: USAID.

UNDESA (United Nations Department of Economic and Social Affairs). 2004. *The Impact of AIDS*. New York: United Nations.

UNICEF (United Nations (International) Children's (Emergency) Fund). 1999. *Children Orphaned by AIDS: Frontline Responses from Eastern and Southern Africa*. New York: UNICEF.

United States Census Bureau. 2002. *The HIV/AIDS Pandemic in the 21st Century*. Washington, DC.

Urdal, Henrik. 2004. 'The Devil in the Demographics: The Effect of Youth Bulges on Domestic Armed Conflict 1950–2000'. *Social Development Papers: Conflict Prevention and Reconstruction* 14. Washington DC: World Bank.

Weiss, Taya. 2004. *Guns in the Borderlands: Reducing the Demand for Small Arms*. Institute of Security Studies Monograph Series 95, January.

Williams, John. 2005. 'Presentation to the US Council on Foreign Affairs', April.

Wilson, Tanya, Sonja Giese, Helen Meintjies, Rhian Croke and Ross Chamberlain. 2002. 'A Conceptual Framework for the Identification, Support and Monitoring of Children Experiencing Orphanhood'. Report published by the HIV/AIDS Programme, Children's Institute, October.

8

Prisons and HIV/AIDS

————•————

Razaan Bailey

Everyone who is detained, including every sentenced prisoner, has the right to conditions of detention that are consistent with human dignity, including at least exercise and the provision, at state expense, of adequate accommodation, nutrition, reading material and medical treatment. (Republic of South Africa Constitution, Section 35 (2) (e))

By entering prisons, prisoners are condemned to imprisonment for their crimes; they should not be condemned to HIV and AIDS. (UNAIDS, WHO and UNICEF 2006, 122)

Introduction

According to the UNAIDS 2006 'Report on the Global AIDS Epidemic', the prevalence of HIV infection in prisons is almost invariably higher than that in the general population. In South Africa, estimates put the figure as high as 41 per cent in the general prison system and even higher in some individual prisons (UNAIDS, WHO and UNICEF 2006, 119). Based on these estimates, it may be that as many as 65 891 out of the 160 712 people incarcerated in South Africa's 240 correctional centres at the end of January 2007 were living with HIV.

Two main factors are likely to lead to high HIV prevalence in prison populations. As K.C. Goyer et al. note, the socio-economic factors that contribute to the spread of HIV are very similar to those that lead to criminal activity and incarceration. They observe that 'the people who are more likely to be in prison are also among the most likely to contract HIV: young, unemployed, un- or under-educated, black men. Many of the socioeconomic factors that place an individual at high risk for contracting HIV, are the same factors which lead to criminal activity and incarceration.' (2006, 6)

For reasons discussed in this chapter, practices within prisons also put prisoners at risk of contracting HIV while incarcerated, which constitutes a violation of prisoners' human rights and is also a public health issue. Offenders are a mobile population and while there is no clear data on recidivism rates in South Africa, some commentators estimate that as many as 85–94 per cent of released prisoners return to prison for repeat offences (Ballington 1998), echoing Michel Foucault's statement that those leaving prison have more chance than before of going back to it (1975). This revolving door between prison and offenders' homes may serve to transmit HIV, as prisoners move between the two communities, both bringing and taking HIV with them. As Goyer et al. go on to argue, 'if their illnesses or infections are not properly treated while in prison, the prisoners will return with these to their communities and may constitute a health risk' (2006, 9).

This chapter examines the factors that put offenders at risk of contracting HIV while imprisoned. While HIV and AIDS do impact on female prisoners, this chapter focuses on men, in order to examine difficult issues of sexual violence and sexual relationships and how these contribute to HIV transmission in prison populations. There is a gender dynamic that underpins these contributing factors to HIV, which replicates many social and cultural beliefs within wider South African society, but which plays out among men in prison (for more on gender issues, see Chapters 2 and 4 in this volume). Specific attention is given to the behaviour of men having sex with men while imprisoned and its role in the transmission of HIV. The chapter concludes by looking at how the Department of Correctional Services (DCS) is dealing with HIV and AIDS and calls for training and capacity-building for the Department, in addition to a more robust effort to mainstream HIV/AIDS management and mitigation programmes in prison populations.

HIV/AIDS in the prison environment

As this chapter demonstrates, sexual violence, tattooing and injecting drug use (IDU) may serve to spread infectious diseases, such as hepatitis, HIV and other sexually transmitted infections (STIs) in prison populations. While these factors also apply to non-prison populations, the risk within prisons is multiplied, as inmates spend all their time in close proximity to each other, largely unobserved, as they negotiate complex power relationships that may expose them to infection.

South Africa has one of the highest prison populations in the world and most inmates are housed in severely overcrowded facilities. The 2006–07 'Annual Report' published by the Judicial Inspectorate of Prisons reveals that average occupancy in the country's prisons is 140 per cent – almost double the number of occupants for which the facilities were designed. The authors calculate that almost three-quarters (72 per cent) of prisons are overcrowded and have a living space per inmate of less than 3.5 m². In the most overcrowded facilities, prisoners often have less than 1.2 m², the size of an average office table, in which they must sleep, eat and spend 23 hours per day (Office of the Inspecting Judge 2007, 16).

In a country where high levels of poverty prevent many arrestees from posting bail, overcrowding is worsened by the often lengthy incarceration of unsentenced prisoners, who may spend anything from four months to three years awaiting trial. In an average month, 18 000–20 000 awaiting-trial detainees are released, usually because the charges against them are withdrawn. Whether an inmate spends one night, one month, or one year in prison, however, he is at risk of being sexually assaulted and contracting HIV and where already living with the virus, adding to the DCS's burden of care.

In compliance with international best practice, the DCS does not conduct mandatory HIV-testing among offenders entering its care. The 2005–06 'Annual Report' of the Judicial Inspectorate of Prisons indicates that natural deaths escalated five-fold between 1996 and 2006, from 1.68 deaths per 1 000 offenders to 9.2 deaths per 1 000 per annum respectively (see Figure 8.1). It also shows that in 2005, 1 507 offenders died of natural causes (Office of the Inspecting Judge 2007, 34).

The 2006–07 'Annual Report' shows that 37 per cent of all deaths occurred within the first 12 months of admission to prison, 52 per cent within the first 24 months and 62 per cent within the first 36 months, indicating that the vast majority of deaths occurred shortly after the prisoners were admitted. This suggests that the majority of prisoners are dying of diseases contracted outside of prison, including HIV/AIDS (Office of the Inspecting Judge 2007, 44). It is impossible to know precisely how many of these deaths are the result of AIDS. As noted by an official DCS spokesperson: 'Research studies to determine the increasing mortality rate and its link with HIV/AIDS have not been undertaken. The causes of death on the [death] certificate are not indicated as HIV/AIDS and it's therefore difficult to directly link it to HIV/AIDS.' ('Prisoners Fight for Life in Court') This reluctance to attribute deaths to AIDS is not unique to either prison populations or South Africa. Given

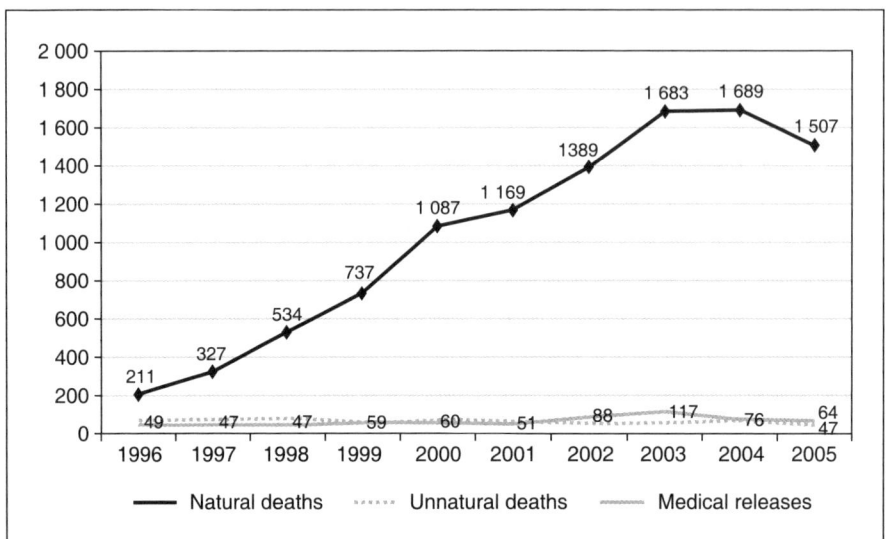

Figure 8.1 Natural and unnatural deaths and medical releases from prisons 1996–2005.

Source: Office of the Inspecting Judge 2007

the stigma still associated with HIV/AIDS, many doctors prefer to record the fatal opportunistic infections (OIs) associated with the virus, which presents a challenge in trying to secure accurate statistics. It is likely, however, that many of these deaths are AIDS-related. The data may in fact underestimate the extent of HIV/AIDS in the prison population, as they exclude those who are sick, those who have yet to show the symptoms of AIDS and offenders who are released on medical parole, in order to allow them to die with dignity. However, the authors of the report believe that the timing of deaths raises serious concerns about the thoroughness of the medical examinations taking place on admission to prison and the quality of medical care provided to prisoners who are admitted with chronic illnesses and in need of medication.

Prison dynamics: The risk of contracting HIV in prison

Prisons are frequently sites for illicit drug use, unsafe injecting practices, tattooing with contaminated equipment, physical and sexual violence, and unprotected sex, which all increase the risk of infection in prison populations. While not a focus of this chapter, features of the prison environment, including overcrowding, often poor nutrition, limited access to healthcare and high rates of airborne and bloodborne diseases may also hasten and exacerbate the onset of AIDS among those already living with HIV (UNAIDS, WHO and UNICEF 2006, 119).

Illicit drug use

IDU in South African correctional centres appears less common than in many other countries, where the sharing of non-sterile equipment has been a major contributing factor to the number of new HIV cases, but the available evidence suggests that levels of IDU are higher than in the general population.

It is impossible to compare directly IDU in prison and civilian populations, but data on more general drug use provide an indication of possible trends. In a national survey conducted by the Nelson Mandela Children's Fund in 2005, only 2.1 per cent of respondents had used cannabis, while less than 1 per cent had used cocaine and sedatives, amphetamines, inhalants, opiates and hallucinogens. Only 4.7 per cent of respondents reported having used injected drugs (Nelson Mandela Children's Fund/HSRC 2005, 74).[1] However, in a survey of arrestees conducted by the Medical Research Council (MRC) and the Institute for Security Studies (ISS) in 1999 and 2002, almost half (47 per cent) of the 2 859 respondents tested positive for one or more of six drugs, including cannabis, mandrax, cocaine, opiates, amphetamines and benzodiazepines (Leggett 2002, 21). With the exception of cannabis, all of these drugs can be injected, indicating that many prisoners entering prison may have used, and will try again to use injected drugs. Given the illegality of drugs, however, clean needles are likely to be in short supply, suggesting that the risk of contracting HIV through the use of contaminated needles is relatively high in prison populations.

Tattooing

Tattooing is prevalent among prisoners. It is part of the extremely powerful gang structure within prisons and tattoos signal belonging to a particular gang. While this is normally a low-risk activity in the broader community, this is not the case in prison. As in the case of IDU, tattooing is not condoned by the correctional authorities and prisoners use whatever sharp implements are at their disposal. These are seldom sterile and are used by many people: 'The inmates use home-made tools for the procedure, either a bit of metal, or even a spoon, that has been sharpened to a point which is able to cut the skin. Tattooing is against the regulations in prison, so a prisoner is not likely to seek medical attention for an infected wound resulting from a tattoo.' (Goyer 2003, 32)

Physical and sexual violence

The levels of violence in South Africa's correctional centres have been extensively documented. According to the DCS, the majority of offenders are imprisoned for aggressive crimes. Of the 160 712 offenders detained at the end of January 2007, a total of 87 369 had committed violent crimes (Office of the Inspecting Judge 2007). It is hardly surprising that the violent behaviour that puts so many people into prison continues there.

The Jali Commission report on prison corruption identifies prison gangs as being responsible for most of this violence. According to the Commission's findings, 'Violence serves three purposes in prisons: firstly, it makes inmates into men rather than boys, secondly, it is used to patrol the boundaries of gang space against warders and thirdly it divides inmates into men and women' (2006, 15). The latter is supported by research conducted by the Centre for the Study of Violence and Reconciliation (CSVR), which found that sexual violence is connected to specific gender relationships that exist in the prison environment. As the authors observe, 'in a social system where manhood is defined by the ability to use violence, a person who cannot fight or will not fight is unable to prove his manliness and is consequently positioned as a woman' (Gear and Nguni 2002, 21). In many cases, violence is associated with rape and unprotected sex (Niehaus 2002).

Sexual relationships among male offenders

As in non-prison populations, many prisoners engage in sexual activity. In some cases these relationships are consensual, but as in correctional facilities worldwide, many prisoners are forced into sex. Those entering custody for the first time often experience some form of violence, such as violent intimidation, coercion, sexual assault and theft when they arrive (Koch and Wood 2002).

The study by the CSVR on sexual activities among male offenders describes how sexual violence and sexual relationships occur within South Africa's correctional centres (Gear and Nguni 2002). It points to the high levels of sexual violence in prison and highlights how a particular understanding of gender maintains these relationships. The study found that prisoners' participation in sexual activity is not usually related to their sexual orientation outside prison, but is rather a product of circumstances in the prison environment. Unlike soldiers in the military, who may have sexual relationships with local women while posted away from home,[2] men in prison turn to one another for a variety of sexual relationships and in many cases, these relationships provide a channel through which destructive notions of what it means to be a man or a woman are generated and exacerbated (Gear and Nguni 2002).

Reflections from the CSVR study

The study highlights three key types of prison sexual relationships: marriage, *uchincha ipondo* ('a pound for a pound') and other consensual relationships. Little information was gathered about the last category, but the study showed that these relationships are defined by feelings of 'love' that partners have for each other. As is the case internationally, however, it is difficult to obtain detailed information about consensual same-sex relationships within prison, as homophobia within the prison environment may lead to victimisation.

'Marriages' are traditionally associated with prison gangs,[3] particularly the gang known as 'the 28s', and are typically structured around a single superior 'husband' who owns and controls one or more 'wives'. The 'wife's' role is to keep the 'home' and service the sexual needs of the 'husband'. It is the 'husband' who penetrates the 'wife'. These 'wives' are from the ranks of the younger males and the relationship is created through a series of manipulative acts when they first enter prison: 'Moves resembling gestures of friendship and entailing offers or provision of food or small luxuries are the most commonly reported form . . . Although the target is frequently unaware, an exchange is taking place and a debt being created for which he will later be expected to pay with sex.' (Gear and Nguni 2002, 18) The relationship between the 'husband' and his 'wife', or 'wives', is usually not consensual, but it does offer some security, as 'wives' obtain the protection of the gang.

Uchincha ipondo describes sexual acts that occur through mutual agreement. Neither of the partners is dominant and the parties come together purely to meet each other's sexual needs. Each partner has an opportunity to penetrate the other. One of the respondents in the study described it in the following way: 'It's mostly young guys who are experimenting with sex . . . and it will be mostly a mutual kind of thing. You find two young guys who do each other favours . . . You'd have one time the one acting as a man and then the other time, the other one swopping . . . They call it 'exchange' (*ipondo*).' (Gear and Nguni 2002, 52) Because *uchincha ipondo* is based on mutual exchange, it is primarily seen as a homosexual activity and thus something that should be punished. As the study's authors note: 'Because *uchincha ipondo* subverts the rules of sex in prison . . . it disallows the allocation of a single gender-status to the protagonists. In so doing, the practice undermines the construction of a masculinity defined by power and penetration, and at the same time interferes with the heterosexually-orientated environment that is the preserve of the gangs.' (Gear and Nguni 2002, 54)

Respondents reported that 'wives' often engage in acts of *uchincha ipondo* with one another. These acts are seen as a way for 'wives' to reclaim their masculinity. There is little information about the use of condoms in these relationships, but given both the circumstances in which sex takes place and the general lack of access to condoms, it is doubtful that they are commonly used. Forced sexual relationships provide few opportunities to negotiate condom use (assuming they are available), to discuss a partner's sexual history, or to find out about their health. Moreover, as in the outside community, even those involved in consensual relationships may frequently be either unwilling or unable to negotiate condom use.

It is well documented, most recently in the findings by the Jali Commission (2006, 29), that many correctional officers turn a blind eye to these sexual activities and that some correctional officers play an active role in facilitating and maintaining them. These findings underscore the importance of prison staff's attitude in ensuring the safety of all prisoners and in creating an environment where prisoners are able to approach staff for help. These attitudes are, in turn, underpinned both by their belief systems and the culture in which they work, suggesting that the DCS needs to actively engage in creating an environment more conducive to protecting prisoners from sexual violence.

More generally, stopping violence in prison and creating safe and respectful environments will require addressing woefully high inmate-to-staff ratios, training staff to identify and respond to violence and more effective surveillance and security measures. It will also require establishing and enforcing appropriate disciplinary sanctions, as well as providing meaningful activities for prisoners.

The changing role of the DCS: A brief history

Prior to the democratic elections in South Africa in 1994, the prison service was run as a militaristic institution. Rather than achieving the goal of transforming offenders into law-abiding citizens, the focus was on punishment. Some experts contend that the focus on punishment failed to rehabilitate prisoners and instead increased recidivism and strengthened criminality: prisons became breeding grounds for gang recruitment and activities.

After 1994, this stringent punitive approach was replaced by one that focused on the rehabilitation and reintegration of offenders into society. This change was influenced by the *Correctional Services Act 111 of 1998* and the 2004 White Paper on Corrections in South Africa. Both of these pieces of legislation have guided the transformation of the DCS and emphasise the importance of creating an environment that recognises the humanity of offenders through the provision of safe custody and rehabilitation. In this vein, the *Correctional Services Act* argues that the DCS should contribute to maintaining and protecting a just, peaceful and safe society by:

- enforcing sentences of the courts in the manner prescribed (by the Act);
- detaining all prisoners in safe custody whilst ensuring their human dignity; and
- promoting the social responsibility and human development of all prisoners and persons subject to community corrections. (*Correctional Services Act 111 of 1998*, section 2)

The White Paper on Corrections acknowledges that while a person is in its custody, the DCS is responsible for providing access to healthcare and that 'this health care should be consistent with that provided by the state to other citizens' (Section 10.7.1, 79). Section 10.8.4 of the White Paper also acknowledges a need for correctional programmes to reduce the impact of HIV and AIDS.

The DCS's response to HIV/AIDS

The DCS's approach to dealing with HIV and AIDS has improved remarkably since the early 1990s, when the Department screened detainees entering prison and kept HIV-positive inmates isolated from the rest of the prison population. This policy came under scrutiny in the mid-1990s following the publication of the World Health Organisation's (WHO) 'Guidelines on HIV Infection and AIDS in Prisons' (1993), which condemned segregation and the DCS subsequently amended its 1996 policy to provide a more rights-conscious framework for tackling HIV/AIDS in the prison population (Goyer 2003).

The revised policy forbids segregation and non-voluntary testing. In order to try to prevent HIV transmission in prisons, it advocates extensive HIV/AIDS education and counselling for inmates and staff, and encourages all prison staff to adopt appropriate safety measures to prevent infection by potentially infected body fluids (Goyer 2003). As well as the policy amendment paper, a separate policy document was circulated to provincial commissioners, relating to the distribution of condoms to prisoners. The new policy called for condoms to be 'provided to the prison population on the same basis as condoms provided in the community' (cited in Goyer 2003, 53).

To date, the DCS HIV and AIDS policy has involved five key interventions: placing condoms in accessible places; providing voluntary counselling to affected offenders; exposing offenders to awareness programmes; treatment of offenders for OIs and STIs and taking steps to start issuing immune-boosting food items. The Department has also recently approved plans to provide antiretroviral (ARV) treatment to offenders. However, this policy has not yet been implemented fully and its overall effectiveness remains uncertain.

Condom distribution

The DCS has, at the policy level, embraced the provision of condoms to inmates. In 2002, the Department stipulated that condoms should be made available in all prisons through the placement of dispensers in common areas. However, condom provision has been inconsistent and influenced by the attitudes of local prison staff, many of whom do not wish to be seen as condoning sexual activities among offenders. Moreover, while placing dispensers in public areas helps to make condoms more accessible, it may also deter prisoners from using them, as they do not want to be identified as having sex. This is partly because of the prohibition on sexual activity and partly due to the stigma of being seen as homosexual. Providing condoms through healthcare services is also problematic, given that these sites are usually very visible in public spaces.

Even when prisoners obtain condoms, they may not use them correctly, or perceive consistent condom use as either desirable or possible within their relationships. Goyer also notes that the condoms available in prisons may not protect inmates from infection through anal sex. During her study in Durban-Westville Medium B prison in KwaZulu-Natal in 2000 and 2001, health staff reported that the condoms provided break during anal intercourse. The condoms are issued by the Department of Health (DoH) and are the same as those provided in the general community, but are designed for vaginal, rather than anal sex (2003).

Access issues and the reluctance of some authorities to distribute condoms are not unique to either South Africa or the prison service. Disseminating condoms and ensuring that they are used correctly and consistently is one of the greatest challenges facing HIV/AIDS prevention programmes the world over. However, these problems point to an urgent need for the DCS to reassess its position on sexual activity in prisons and suggest the need for additional, less public sites for condom distribution, as well as the distribution of more durable condoms.

HIV/AIDS awareness and prevention

The DCS has conducted HIV/AIDS awareness training among both inmates and DCS staff, with activities in each province co-ordinated by a provincial HIV/AIDS co-ordinator (PHC). The PHC is identified as a member of the nursing staff in each province whose duties include: advising Commanders and heads of prisons on the implementation of HIV/AIDS programmes and policies, monitoring the efficiency of STI clinics in all the prisons in the province and implementing the Department's HIV/AIDS policy (Goyer 2003).

In the 2005–06 financial year, the Department's activities were boosted with the provision of US$600 000 (R3.6 million) for HIV and AIDS activities from the US Presidential Emergency Plan for AIDS Relief (PEPFAR). This funding continued into the 2006–07 financial year. With assistance from PEPFAR and others, the DCS conducted 35 400 awareness sessions on HIV/AIDS in the 2005–06 financial year and 47 438 in the 2006–07 financial year (DCS 2006, 31; 2007). These sessions included discussions and lectures on HIV/AIDS, as well as on other health promotion topics. According to the DCS website, offenders are also exposed to positive HIV/AIDS messaging through participation in events such as World AIDS Day and International Candle Light Memorial Day (DCS n.d.).

Community agencies have taken the lead in providing awareness and support services. Many DCS staff report feeling that they are inadequately trained to address HIV/AIDS-related issues and have generally welcomed these initiatives. However, DCS personnel who work with prisoners 24 hours a day, seven days a week are best placed to create an HIV/AIDS-sensitive environment. These critically important individuals need training, support and appropriate supervision to enable them to carry out their HIV/AIDS-related duties with professionalism and confidence.

In addition to formal training sessions, the DCS is implementing a peer education programme among its staff and inmates. An example of such an intervention being offered in the correctional environment is the Themba HIV/AIDS intervention in Boksburg Correctional Centre, which is facilitated by young people from similar backgrounds to those in custody. The peer educators, while living outside the correctional facility, speak the same language (including current street slang) and understand and take into account local circumstances, ethics and cultural values. In 2005–06, 1 254 offenders were trained as peer educators, while in 2006–07, 1 159 DCS officials were trained as master trainers and peer educators (DCS 2006, 2007).

Despite these promising initiatives, questions remain about the reach of the DCS programme and the extent of its responsibility in trying to encourage positive behaviour changes. Given the high levels of recidivism in South Africa, activities in the prison environment should arguably be linked to ongoing infrastructures in offenders' home communities. On release from custody, a male prisoner may be motivated to make changes in his life or maintain those made in prison. However, without support from others – particularly affirming peer and social networks – he may find it difficult to implement these changes. In order to be effective, HIV-prevention strategies must help prisoners to build peer networks in and outside of prison that promote, support and reinforce harm reduction and behaviour changes. These are long-term interventions and, as long as young men continue to pass through the revolving door between prison and outside communities, they will need long-term support to undertake less risky sexual and drug-taking behaviours.

Testing and treatment

The provision of ARV therapy to HIV-positive prisoners has been a source of considerable debate and controversy. While addressing the epidemic has been a long-standing concern in the DCS, until recently, much of the discussion on the issue occurred outside of the public domain. This changed in 2006, when an urgent court application was brought against the Department by fifteen offenders from the Westville Prison in KwaZulu-Natal. The involvement of high-profile civil society groups, such as the Treatment Action Campaign (TAC) and the Aids Law Project (ALP), helped to highlight the issue of treating offenders in the public domain. The court ordered the DCS to provide immediate access to ARV therapy for all sentenced prisoners. While this was not the first time that the DCS had been ordered by the court to provide ARV treatment, the Westville case powerfully illustrated the power of civil society institutions to influence the judiciary, as well as the broader reluctance of the government to take command of the HIV/AIDS crisis.

The DoH is responsible for the provision of ARVs through its 'Comprehensive HIV and AIDS Care, Management and Treatment Plan', with prisons identified as one of several treatment sites. The Grootvlei Correctional Centre was the first site accredited to provide ARV therapy (DCS 2006, 31). The 2006–07 'Annual Report' identifies eight additional correctional centres to be accredited as Comprehensive Prevention, Treatment, Care and Support Centres. The identified sites are: Pietermaritzburg, Durban-Westville Medium B, Qalakabusha, St Albans Medium B, Johannesburg Medium C, Kroonstad Medium C, Groenpunt and Kimberley correctional centres (DCS 2007, 15).

However, as is the case outside of the prison system, there have been delays in the accreditation of these correctional centres into treatment sites. In compliance with the court order, however, the DCS has facilitated access to treatment by transporting offenders to the nearest accredited public health centres. There are currently 2 323 offenders receiving treatment, while 18 585 offenders have undergone voluntary counselling and testing (DCS 2007).

The DCS has begun a process of up-skilling its health staff in order to respond more effectively to the needs of offenders living with HIV/AIDS. In the 2005–06 financial year, for example, 147 correctional officers were trained in voluntary counselling and testing, while 37 healthcare workers were given training on how to administer and interpret rapid HIV/AIDS test kits (DCS 2006). The Department also participated in the formulation and arrangement of a national contract for the issue of immune-boosting food items (DCS n.d.).

Conclusion

This chapter is limited in that it has not explored the deeper questions of the meaning behind the activities and relationships discussed, nor the push and pull of environmental factors, or the question of prison staff and HIV. Instead, it has sought to illuminate the links between sexual violence, prison culture and high-risk sexual behaviour in South Africa's prisons. While there have been some useful studies on these links to HIV transmission, knowledge about the gendered dynamics of male prisoner vulnerability to HIV have not been widely discussed within policy circles.

The brief overview of the key components of the DCS's response to HIV/AIDS shows that over the last decade, the Department has made significant progress in trying to reduce the spread and effects of the epidemic in the prison population. However, there are still areas of weakness, particularly the Department's contradictory policy standpoints on sexual activity among prisoners and the implications for condom-dissemination programmes. The discomfort experienced by DCS personnel when called upon to engage in HIV/AIDS issues also suggests that emphasis must remain on training and capacity-building within the service. Correctional services staff are most strategically placed to address HIV/AIDS issues, but they can only do this if they are provided with the skills and human and financial resources to do so.

Most importantly, the issue of HIV/AIDS needs to be mainstreamed: it cannot be meaningfully addressed if it is simply tacked on to the range of duties already expected of often overstretched personnel. Addressing HIV/AIDS must be integrated into all aspects of DCS work: correctional officers must be supported to address HIV/AIDS and performance on HIV/AIDS indicators should become part of the Department's evaluation criteria. Building capacity and a system more sensitive to the epidemic will take time and resources, suggesting greater scope for both short-term and longer-term partnerships with civil society and private institutions involved in training, counselling, care and support.

Notes

1. For more information on IDU and HIV and measures to address the transmission of HIV through IDU, visit the International Harm Reduction Association website at http://www.ihra.net.
2. This does not mean that the possibility of spreading or becoming infected with HIV is not present.
3. Over the past 100 years, gangs have become institutionalised in prisons. The dominant gangs in South Africa are the 26s, 27s and 28s. For an understanding of how these gangs operate, see Steinberg 2004.

References

Ballington, J. 1998. *Punishment in South Africa*. Masters thesis, University of the Witwatersrand.
DCS (Department of Correctional Services). n.d. 'Making a Difference in HIV and AIDS'. Available at http://www.dcs.gov.za, accessed 10 December 2007.

————. 2006. 'Annual Report for the 2005/06 Financial Year'. Government of South Africa.

————. 2007. 'Annual Report for the 2006/07 Financial Year'. Government of South Africa.

Foucault, Michel. 1975. *Discipline and Punishment: The Birth of the Prison*. New York: Random House.

Gear, Sasha and Kindiza Nguni. 2002. *DAAI DING: Sex, Sexual Violence and Coercion in Men's Prisons*. Braamfontein: CSVR.

Goyer, K.C. 2003. *HIV/AIDS in Prisons: Problems, Policies and Potential*. Institute for Security Studies Monograph Series 79, February. Available at http://www.iss.co.za/Pubs/Monographs/No79/Chap1.pdf, accessed 18 June 2006.

Goyer, K.C., Yusuf Saloojee, Marlise Richter and Chloe Hardy. 2006. 'HIV/AIDS in Prison: Treatment, Intervention, and Reform'. Unpublished submission to the Jali Commission, November.

Jali Commission. 2006. 'Final Report of the Jali Commission'. Available at http://www.dcs.gov.za/Documents/Jali/JALI%20Commission.pdf, accessed 5 November 2006.

Koch, Ros and Catherine Wood. 2002. *Case Studies of Children with Experience of the Criminal Justice System in South Africa*. Cape Town: Institute of Criminology, University of Cape Town.

Leggett, Ted (ed.). 2002. *Drugs and Crime in South Africa*. Institute for Security Studies Monograph Series 69, March.

Nelson Mandela Children's Fund/HSRC (Human Sciences Research Council). 2005. *South African National HIV Prevalence, HIV Incidence, Behaviour and Communication Survey, 2005*. Pretoria: HSRC Press.

Niehaus, Isak. 2002. 'Renegotiating Masculinity in the South African Lowveld: Narratives of Male-Male Sex in Labour Compounds and in Prisons'. *Journal of African Studies* 61(1): 77–97.

Office of the Inspecting Judge. 2007. 'Annual Report 2006/2007'. Tshwane: Judicial Inspectorate of Prisons.

'Prisoners Fight for Life in Court', 18 April 2006. Available at http://www.iafrica.com/pls/cms/iac, accessed 22 June 2006.

Steinberg, Johnny. 2004. *The Number*. Cape Town: Jonathan Ball.

UNAIDS (Joint United Nations Programme on HIV/AIDS). 2006. 'Report on the Global AIDS Epidemic'. May, UNAIDS/06.20E.

UNAIDS (Joint United Nations Programme on HIV/AIDS), WHO (World Health Organisation) and UNICEF (United Nations (International) Children's (Emergency) Fund. 2006. 'Report on the Global AIDS Epidemic'. Geneva: UNAIDS.

WHO (World Health Organisation). 1993. 'Guidelines on HIV Infection and AIDS in Prisons'. Available at http://www.data.unaids.org/Publications/IRC-pub01/JC277-WHO-Guidel-Prisons_en.pdf, accessed 23 March 2008.

9

The Military Sector and HIV/AIDS

Angela Ndinga-Muvumba[1]

Our young members believe that the SANDF can only go to war with a living, breathing and bleeding enemy. Well, that is the kind of enemy our grandfathers went to war with, but we now live in a new world where poverty and disease kill more people than people who die in countries at war with each other. AIDS, coupled with poverty, will single-handedly wipe out an entire family. So who is the enemy now? (Vuthela 2005, 26)

Introduction

How will South African state security institutions effectively address HIV/AIDS? The South African National Defence Force (SANDF) has openly stated that if the HIV/AIDS epidemic in its ranks is not urgently addressed, combat readiness will be compromised and the defence force will not be able to fulfil its mandate (SAMHS 2005, 2).[2] Under the direction and management of its health services wing – the South African Military Health Services (SAMHS) – the defence force carries out HIV/AIDS prevention, treatment and clinical research through two major programmes. The first of these is Masibambisane ('Beyond Awareness'), a prevention campaign designed to raise awareness among the SANDF's troops, their families and their communities. The second is Project Phidisa, a SANDF-managed clinical research programme that seeks to generate new knowledge about the challenges of managing antiretroviral (ARV) treatment.

The strategic response to HIV/AIDS by conventional security actors has been under-researched. This chapter examines the South African military's programmes for the management and mitigation of HIV/AIDS and draws on some of the literature about African militaries and the debates about HIV/AIDS as a security threat to the defence forces. Due to limited space and because others cover these issues elsewhere (see, for example, Chapter 3), this chapter does not seek to address the South African government's response to HIV/AIDS in the civilian sector, nor many of the vital underlying social and medical debates about treatment and prevention. The main focus is an exploration of the SANDF's response to the epidemic and questions about the security dimensions of HIV/AIDS within state security institutions. This chapter also briefly addresses issues of human and traditional security and concludes by exploring how these concepts – within the context of HIV/AIDS – relate to the priorities of a traditional security pillar, such as the military, and its response to the epidemic.

The evolving role of African militaries

African militaries emerged from colonialism and apartheid as symbolic actors in the task of building new African states. This post-colonial legacy cannot be underestimated. As Martin Rupiya has noted in a review of southern African militaries, 'the armed forces are seen not only as an instrument to address security concerns, but also as a concrete national symbol that represents and participates in ceremonies which confirm the status of the new nation' (2005, 1). In southern Africa, for example, liberation movements in Angola, Mozambique, Namibia and South Africa have all established priorities for integrating their defence forces into nation-building (2005, 367–71).

Moreover, there is a new and urgent role for Africa's militaries beyond their national borders. The inevitable consequences of underdevelopment and authoritarian regimes in parts of Africa have undermined peace and stability on the continent. A simple assessment of United Nations (UN) peacekeeping missions demonstrates that the continent is still very much dependent on such operations to maintain and build peace. Out of 90 000 peacekeepers in the world in 2006, nearly 58 346 of the UN's military and civilian police were in Africa (UN Department of Peacekeeping Operations n.d.). Article 13 of the African Union (AU) Peace and Security Council's Protocol calls for the establishment of an African Standby Force (ASF) by 2010 (2002). The ASF – consisting of standby brigades in central, southern, eastern, North and West Africa – will undertake traditional peacekeeping operations, as well as observer missions and peace-building activities. Each of the ASF's regional standby brigades is expected to maintain a force of about 3 000 infantry soldiers, as well as 1 258 logistical specialists, signallers, engineers, military police and civilian support staff for rapid deployment in Africa at appropriate notice (Cilliers and Malan 2005). South Africa will participate in the southern African brigade, which is being marshalled by the Southern African Development Community (SADC).

South Africa's defence force faces the same expectations as other African militaries in terms of nation-building and it has already embraced the new role of peacekeeping. In the southern African context, the symbolic meaning of the military as the embodiment of the state and its liberation from colonial power abounds. The African National Congress (ANC) government, for example, sought to undertake a massive refurbishment of defence weapons and equipment through a strategic defence package deal in 2001, which was estimated to cost R29 billion (approximately US$4 142 857 143) and is reported to have exceeded this amount (Le Roux 2005, 263; Govender 2007, 197–205). New arms for the new South Africa were prioritised, but some criticised the ANC for seeking to increase the defence budget, while other issues, such as poverty, remained a challenge.

At the same time, the government was cognisant of the importance of other roles of the military. Through reform of the apartheid-era force and defence management, the SANDF increased the number of women in service, strengthened civilian oversight and focused on peacekeeping. As a traditional security actor, the SANDF has taken on both traditional and non-traditional priorities and sought to cloak itself in the raiment of military might, while also embracing humanitarianism. Finally, because of HIV/AIDS, this traditional pillar of security has had to look at non-military threats to its capacity, such as gender inequality, which fuels the spread of the virus and poverty, and undermines prevention, treatment and care. The end result is a defence force that is looking *inward* at a threat that is non-military, one that is bound up in social, cultural, economic, historical and gender factors.

HIV/AIDS as a potential threat

Analyses thus far have been largely speculative and unable to address the current status of HIV/AIDS in national armies, its implications for regional conflict management and more broadly, for human security. In the beginning, a series of assumptions about the risk environment of military life and culture, the paucity in HIV/AIDS management and mitigation strategies within defence structures and the secretive and defensive attitude of senior-level military officials and gatekeepers to externally led HIV/AIDS studies resulted in impressionistic analyses and an overemphasis on unsubstantiated data that indicated that HIV/AIDS was much higher in military populations than it actually is (Barnett and Prins 2006; see also Chapter 11 in this volume).

A 1998 UN report noted that soldiers usually have higher rates of sexually transmitted infections (STIs) than civilians. It is true that untreated STIs increase susceptibility to HIV infection. Moreover, the combination of the high-risk profile of soldiers and their heightened susceptibility to HIV seemed to suggest that they were likely to have almost *two to five times higher rates* of HIV than their civilian counterparts (UNAIDS 1998). This has remained largely unproven; even when military populations have higher rates of HIV than civilians, researchers have not yet been able to provide evidence from enough militaries to prove a pattern. The US-based Council on Foreign Relations issued a report in July 2005 that noted, however, that in some countries, average HIV prevalence is higher within the defence forces: for example, Botswana's average HIV prevalence was 32.9 per cent in 2000 and the average prevalence for its police and armed forces was approximately 40 per cent. The report also announced prevalence data from Kenya, which had an overall HIV rate of 6.4 per cent among civilians and 9.4 per cent in its military (Garret 2005, 28).

However, age, rank and deployment affect the vulnerability of soldiers. In some countries, young recruits have lower HIV rates than civilians because they do not have the money to pay for sex workers or are restricted to military bases. Between 1999 and 2000, the Ethiopian Defence Forces (EDF) mobilised troops to fight in the Ethiopian-Eritrean war and conducted mandatory HIV screening on some of its new recruits. The results demonstrated an urban/rural variation in HIV prevalence: 7.2 per cent of urban recruits tested positive, while only 3.8 per cent of recruits from rural areas were HIV-positive. Finally, a group of retired soldiers recently remobilised to fight in the war with Eritrea were also tested for HIV. This group of 12 553 had an HIV prevalence of 23 per cent, suggesting that older soldiers who had been reintegrated into the civilian population could have higher rates of HIV (Berhe, Gemechu and De Waal 2005).

There is some evidence from West Africa that involvement in peacekeeping can increase HIV prevalence. Nigerian peacekeepers returning from the Economic Community of West Africa's Ceasefire Monitoring Group (ECOMOG) missions in Liberia and Sierra Leone during the 1990s had nearly twice as high infection rates as non-peacekeepers. The Lagos-based Medical Command School Headquarters found that the overall HIV prevalence among Nigerian troops had increased dramatically during the period of the ECOMOG interventions. In 1989, HIV prevalence in the Nigerian army was less than 1 per cent. By 1997 prevalence had climbed to 5 per cent and by 1999, to approximately 10 per cent. Moreover, the risk of HIV infection increased dramatically for each year spent on deployment in these conflict zones. After one year of deployment, the average risk of infection was 7 per cent. Within three years of service, the risk of HIV infection for the average soldier had increased to 15 per cent (Adefalolu 1999, 201–18).

Beyond this, what are the ramifications of high levels of HIV/AIDS for military planning, recruitment and deployment? Analysts have expounded on several possible impacts: a heavy toll on the decision-making command structure, rising costs in retraining highly skilled personnel, delayed deployment to international peace operations and competition for resources with the civilian sector, in order to meet the demands of expensive HIV/AIDS treatment. An additional concern is the vulnerability of peacekeepers to HIV in conflict zones and the risk of these troops spreading the virus among civilian populations at home and abroad. In the end, many of these impacts have either been carefully concealed by militaries or pre-empted through strategic planning by many of the world's defence forces. Many scholars and experts now argue that it is not clear whether HIV has (or could have) a damaging effect on the military's capabilities (see, for example, De Waal 2006), while others call for more holistic and integrated studies over a longer period of time. Ultimately, the fact remains that it is not yet clear how HIV/AIDS is impacting on militaries. While many military establishments have acknowledged that HIV/AIDS is increasing their disease burden, the impact on strategic planning, recruitment and deployment remains a mystery.

The new South African defence force

Since South Africa's first democratic elections in 1994, the SANDF's core evolution has centred on transforming its force membership, becoming a fully professional defence force that reflects the diversity of South Africa and enhancing its capacity to contribute to peace-support operations and other duties (Le Roux and Boshoff 2005, 183). The South African Department of Defence (DoD) is made up of the Defence Secretariat and the SANDF, which was established in April 1994, in accordance with South Africa's interim Constitution of 1993. The SANDF is composed of an army, navy, air force and military health services. Immediately following the 1994 elections, the government embarked on a process of integration and transformation of the old South African Defence Force (SADF).

At the centre of transformation was a perception that the new country's defence forces should contribute to the post-apartheid government's *raison d'être*: empowerment, reconciliation and nation-building (Le Roux 2005). In many ways, a premium was placed upon changing the hearts and minds of South African soldiers and freedom fighters. The new military would be a reflection of the Rainbow Nation: multiracial, multilingual and multicultural. It would respond to insecurity by preventing conflict and aim to provide service from a people-centred perspective by supporting the pillars of a peaceful, democratic society. Consequently, the DoD's immediate post-apartheid evolution was circumscribed by the process of integrating combatants from the liberation armies, the establishment of accountability mechanisms to civil authority, and aligning defence policy to international law and the challenges of the post-cold-war era's new demands for peacekeeping capacity in Africa.

Each of these three foci has seen a mixture of success and failure. Scholars and experts, such as Len le Roux, have addressed these issues elsewhere (see, for example, Le Roux 2005; Le Roux and Boshoff 2005). What is most important to note is that the new military has been in a state of constant transformation. First, by 1998, the process of integration had brought together approximately 82 724 former members of the SADF, troops from the defence forces of Transkei, Bophuthatswana, Venda and Ciskei (TBVC), cadres of the African National Congress' (ANC) armed wing, Umkhonto weSizwe (MK) and the Azanian People's Liberation Army (APLA), and fighters from the Inkatha Freedom Party's (IFP) KwaZulu Self-Protection Forces (Le Roux and Boshoff 2005, 179; SANDF 1998, 70). The integration process was charged with political tensions. At the point of integration, the SADF's size and structure dominated the other forces. In 1998, there were 57 053 SADF soldiers, compared with a combined total of 24 482 personnel from the other forces. The period of integration and transformation led to significant changes in the composition of the SANDF. With more than 10 000 new recruits and retrenchment or retirement of SADF and other soldiers, by 2003 the defence force was 62 per cent black, 1 per cent Asian, 12 per cent coloured and 25 per cent white. An estimated 79 per cent of SANDF members were male and 21 per cent female (SANDF 1998, 71; DoD '2002–03 Annual Report' cited in Le Roux 2005, 254–55). Today's force is an estimated 70 000.

Second, under the 1996 Constitution of South Africa, it was established that the SANDF would be focused on defending the country from a number of traditional, as well as new threats. The new military would not only be responsible for defending South Africa's sovereignty and territorial integrity, it could also be called upon to provide maintenance or essential services and support to 'any department of state for the purpose of socio-economic upliftment' (cited in Le Roux 2005, 242). The DoD's White Paper of the period between 1994 and 1996 places a strategic emphasis on planning for co-operation with other states and on conflict management, prevention and resolution (cited in Le Roux 2005, 256).

By 2003, the SANDF had deployed almost 700 peacekeepers to Burundi and 150 specialists to the UN's peace operation in the Democratic Republic of the Congo (DRC) (Global Defence 2003). Indeed, despite technical, logistical, budgetary and human resource constraints, the South African government has demonstrated a remarkable commitment to peacekeeping in Africa. By 2005, South Africa had not only deployed 3 000 troops to the continent's most troubled countries, but also galvanised support for initiatives such as the AU and its plans for the ASF (Le Roux 2005, 261). The SANDF also engaged in policing during the immediate post-apartheid era, as a service to support the police services. Furthermore, 3 000 SANDF members were engaged in border control and rural protection activities in 2004 (Le Roux 2005, 263).

Having completed its initial period of transition, the DoD intends to carry out strategic planning and modifications to cope with new international and domestic demands. Experts within the defence department have concluded that the new South African military must address evolving and unanticipated demands at home and abroad. The South African government's commitment to peace in Africa will require future engagement in conflict management and peace support operations. Africa's new security architecture will demand sustained engagement and expertise. Finally, rising rates of crime inside South Africa require the SANDF's continued support to the police.

The SANDF's response to HIV/AIDS

In 2002, nearly half of HIV-positive southern Africans were South African (Nattrass 2002, 2). South Africa is the largest investor in sub-Saharan Africa and yet its wealth relative to the rest of the continent has not enabled it to escape the HIV/AIDS pandemic (UNAIDS 2006, 6; see also Chapter 2 in this volume for an explanation of the historical, political and social factors that have fuelled the epidemic in South Africa). A 2005 study published by the Joint United Nations Programme on HIV/AIDS (UNAIDS) and the World Health Organisation (WHO) reported that among people aged fifteen and older, an increased death rate of 62 per cent was experienced between 1997 and 2002.

As part of the March 2006 survey by Tony Barnett and Gwyn Prins for UNAIDS on HIV/AIDS and security, senior military officers from African countries were asked if they knew of any AIDS deaths in their services. The South African response was: 'No.' Certainly this response was confounding. In July 2004, Minister of Defence, Mosiuoa Lekota reported that 17 500 of the 70 000 members of the force were infected with HIV (Hosken 2004; Michaels 2004). How could it be, then, that the South African military leadership could deny AIDS deaths in the services? South Africa bears the greatest AIDS burden in the world, yet the scale of the epidemic and its toll on its most sensitive and privileged institutions remains guarded (Barnett and Prins 2006, 53).

The impact of HIV/AIDS on the SANDF

Despite the silence about AIDS deaths, the SANDF has openly stated that if HIV/AIDS is not urgently addressed, the epidemic will have a negative impact on its combat readiness and the defence force will not be able to fulfil its mandate (SAMHS 2005, 2). It is important to note that the DoD, the military's Surgeon-General and other sectors of the SANDF structure have not expanded on this statement. Of equal importance in a balanced analysis is the overwhelming view of most experts – despite previous assertions – that it is quite possible that the HIV epidemic in the SANDF reflects that of South Africa's general population, no more and no less. Indeed, the SANDF has stated: 'The HIV epidemic in the SANDF seems to mirror that of the general population. This is contrary to the popular view that military populations could have an HIV prevalence that is 2–5 times higher than civilian populations in peacetime, and up to 100 times higher during war according to UNAIDS and the international Civil Military Alliance.' (SAMHS 2005–06)

Officially and publicly, HIV prevalence in the South African military hovered at 17 per cent and the HIV incidence rate was approximately 0.19 per cent per year. This information was drawn from a sample of more than 10 per cent of the total SANDF population in March 2000 (SAMHS 2005, 1; 2005–06). SAMHS has subsequently noted that SANDF HIV prevalence in 2003 – based on the 2000 rate, classified incidence data and surveys performed by the South African Department of Health (DoH) – could be around 23 per cent (SAMHS 2005, 1; 2005–06).

The role of SAMHS

SAMHS is composed of approximately 8 000 doctors, nurses, social workers and other healthcare professionals and is led by the SANDF's Surgeon-General, Lieutenant-General Vejaynand Indurjith Ramlakan.[3] Members of the military health service are deployed domestically and abroad. These men and women are part of the AU's mission to the Comoros, the Darfur region of Sudan and other external deployments. They are responsible for coping with HIV/AIDS and other physical, psychological and mental threats to successful operations (SAMHS News 2006).

The history of military medicine is critical to understanding the new challenges facing SAMHS as a result of the HIV/AIDS epidemic. Military medicine is designed to ensure that militaries are able to carry out their overall missions and to sustain the force, its readiness, its strength and its projection capability. Military health has thus focused on maintaining health in peace and on the collection, diagnosis, evacuation and treatment of the sick and wounded in war. Other functions – to provide dental, psychological and general care, and to procure and maintain medical equipment and expertise – have evolved in tandem with the development of medical and scientific knowledge. The medical personnel in this profession are soldiers and trained and linked to the doctrine of their military.

Military health services are established to reduce disease burdens of armies in order to ensure that their missions are complete and successful. The problem with HIV/AIDS for today's militaries is that it is a chronic disease, which presents novel, and as yet unexamined questions for the human rights of soldiers, the role of military medicine and the relationship between militaries and civilian populations. An example of this evolution is that most of Africa's militaries provide care, support, and to a lesser extent, treatment for their soldiers and their families. Given that there is no cure for HIV/AIDS, the response of military health services has had to evolve to address long-term treatment, support and care.

The implicit change is tremendous: HIV-positive members must maintain access to nutrition, psycho-social support and treatment, if they are to live full and productive lives. Under these circumstances, HIV/AIDS has taken military health services to new frontiers. Militaries in Lesotho, Namibia, Tanzania, Zimbabwe and elsewhere in Africa have co-operated with SAMHS to develop strategies for providing home-based care and treatment. Military health personnel from these countries (many of whom have received training from SAMHS)[4] are struggling to unravel the psycho-social and gendered causes of HIV transmission, in order to prevent new infections, and trying to inculcate long-term behaviour changes that address power dynamics. In peace and war, SAMHS has had to take on new roles in order to address the disease burden of HIV/AIDS (CCR 2006).

The SANDF's vulnerability to HIV/AIDS

Four types of vulnerability to HIV/AIDS can be identified: first, each soldier is vulnerable to infection, illness and death. Since members must perform their duties in high-stress and hostile environments, the health and well-being of soldiers is particularly important. If left untreated, HIV/AIDS threatens the fitness and mental alertness of soldiers. Second, the mission of the defence force is vulnerable to the impact of AIDS. The SANDF's military force design is dependent on groups of soldiers functioning as one co-ordinated structure. If members are compromised, the system will fail. Moreover, the loss of key personnel, such as pilots, drivers and signallers, will cost the government in terms of training new personnel and replacements. Third, HIV/AIDS makes the entire defence organisation vulnerable. Individuals – particularly those with exceptional skills and specific experience – are irreplaceable. Senior-ranking officers, in particular, gain their expertise through specific operations. This expertise cannot be completely replaced by training and several analysts have argued that AIDS-related morbidity and mortality in the officer corps may compromise operational effectiveness (see, for example, Rupiya 2006). Finally, the SANDF's increased costs for disease management will impact on the overall defence budget, possibly taking resources from other sectors and priorities (SAMHS 2005, 3).

These vulnerabilities are linked in a chain of cause and consequences. Each soldier's vulnerability impacts on the readiness and success rate of a mission. If a mission loses a soldier to HIV, or if that soldier is unable to carry out his/her duties effectively because of HIV-related illness, the mission experiences greater vulnerability. If, for example, a mission cannot be operationalised because there are too few deployable members, perhaps because they do not meet mandatory health requirements for fitness, the defence organisation's knowledge, skills and resources are weakened. The impact of HIV/AIDS is experienced at the individual level, the level of operations and finally, in long-term institutional consequences. Because HIV/AIDS is a reoccurring event, the defence force is repeatedly vulnerable.

In April 2001, SAMHS launched the SANDF's comprehensive HIV/AIDS management and mitigation programme. Most of Africa's defence forces have instituted similar HIV/AIDS prevention, care, support and treatment programmes (CCR 2005). First, SAMHS responds to HIV/AIDS on a 'continuum of care', whereby prevention, promotion, diagnostics, treatment, rehabilitation, terminal care and research and development are designed to make HIV more manageable for the individual soldier and for the organisation. SAMHS provides services to more than 70 000 SANDF members and the entire DoD (of which 20 per cent are civilians), as well as their nearly 350 000 dependants. SAMHS works in three military hospitals, four military base hospitals, 36 sick-bays, a number of institutes, referral centres and health centres, and 42 military medical health clinics (see SAMHS News 2006).

South Africa's defence structure is striving towards normalising the epidemic. Despite the implementation of specific HIV/AIDS programmes, the DoD and SAMHS have the ultimate goal of treating HIV/AIDS like any other chronic, progressive and potentially life-threatening diseases, such as cancer or tuberculosis (TB). In this respect, the DoD espouses a non-discriminatory HIV/AIDS policy. The aspiration to normalise HIV/AIDS is linked to the defence force's need to build a long-term institutional foundation for comprehensive HIV/AIDS management and mitigation and to reduce the AIDS stigma. The SAMHS approach to HIV/AIDS, nevertheless, still treats the disease as requiring an exceptional response by virtue of the fact that HIV/AIDS requires new approaches through behaviour change communication, counselling and testing and new technologies and research into treatment. SAMHS has two major programmes, which provide HIV/AIDS prevention, care, support and treatment through a clinical research initiative (Lekota 2003).

HIV prevention: 'Beyond Awareness'
Established in 2001, Masibambisane ('Beyond Awareness') is a prevention campaign targeting SANDF management, troops and their families and communities. The programme fosters knowledge about prevention of HIV/AIDS and STIs through education and mass-marketing campaigns. It promotes individual responsibility for staying HIV-negative, as well as voluntary counselling and testing (VCT). Masibambisane implements an HIV-in-the-workplace programme to ensure adequate condom distribution and administers a peer-to-peer education programme that emphasises awareness of HIV and STIs. SAMHS monitors and evaluates the effectiveness of its programme. The health service also updates members of the

military on HIV information and management policies and co-ordinates the military's response to HIV/AIDS. The basic components of the Masibambisane programme are: counselling, psycho-social services and spiritual support, management of STIs, general healthcare, immunisations, nutritional support, provision of post-exposure prophylaxis (PEP) and palliative care.

The programme's originality and most promising strength lie in its efforts to develop unique non-traditional medical interventions. For example, Masibambisane has a 'Moral and Value Enhancement Programme of the Pastoral Services', which teaches and promotes universal ethical values such as honour, integrity, truth and love. Members are trained to think about these values in an integrative manner in behaviour change training and to call upon them when faced with choices about sexual conduct in the field. Masibambisane also has a Gender Equity Project, through the SAMHS Department of Social Work, which is designed to empower women and men to address gender inequality and its relationship with HIV/AIDS. Finally, SAMHS has developed a theatre production and two short films, one of which addresses the problem of alcohol and drug abuse during peacekeeping operations.

There are a number of other innovations. While not all members of the defence force receive the same training, all members are exposed to the prevention messages and psycho-social support of Masibambisane. This is important because it provides the opportunity for members to gain a common culture relating to life skills and issues such as gender inequality and human rights. The members of SANDF receive this information automatically by virtue of joining the army. Unlike regular members of the South African population, they are a captive audience.

Moreover, SAMHS is gaining expertise in other areas, such as co-infection. In December 2005, one of several routine medical tests conducted by SAMHS revealed ten cases of TB. The reported infectious cases received the required treatment to which personnel responded positively. SAMHS has since institutionalised routine health testing for TB and other related opportunistic infections (OIs) (DoD 2006). The SANDF's corporate communication department uses the bulletin *Department of Defence* as an educational tool and strategy to ensure that SANDF personnel are kept abreast of effective measures to prevent new infections.

An area for concern is the long-term sustainability of Masibambisane. The government and the DoD drive the programme, but it relies heavily on external funding – as indeed most of Africa's HIV/AIDS and military programmes do. One reason for normalising HIV treatment and prevention is this need to integrate it into other military health services. It will also be difficult to maintain long-term HIV/AIDS management in the SANDF, as long as there is no ability to measure and evaluate SAMHS's successes and challenges in delivering effective prevention and treatment. Experts within SAMHS have cited the importance of building its research and development capacity, in order to begin measuring the organisation's progress.

Normalising the disease will help to alleviate the enormous burden on a small group of senior officers to manage the programme. While the organisation is training many peer educators within the defence forces, it is clearly overburdened by HIV/AIDS. Furthermore, it is not yet clear how much the DoD's senior management are invested in the SAMHS programme. Although the DoD is in charge of overall leadership, there is as yet no obvious indication that the HIV/AIDS interventions speak to issues beyond health, such as policy-planning and strategic design. It is rare, for example, that strategic planners working within another of the SANDF's forces will take on HIV/AIDS as an issue, or engage in planning for handling the long-term impacts of the disease. Moreover, according to a confidential source in March 2006, other health problems (ranging from heart disease, diabetes, high cholesterol to malaria and TB, depression and substance abuse) also preoccupy SAMHS. Without ownership of HIV/AIDS across the DoD, SAMHS will be constrained in its efforts to normalise, widen and maintain long-term support for HIV/AIDS management and mitigation.

HIV treatment: 'Making Better, Prolonging Life'[5]
Project Phidisa, launched in December 2003, is a SANDF-managed clinical research programme that seeks to generate new knowledge about the challenges of providing ARVs. The clinical research of Phidisa is supported by the US Department of Defence and the US National Institutes of Health (NIH) through the National Institute of Allergy and Infectious Diseases (NIAID) (SANDF 2006). According to its website, Phidisa's three key objectives are to:

1. provide treatment to qualifying HIV-positive SANDF members and their dependants at six selected research locations;
2. answer research questions relevant to South Africa on the use of ARV therapy in the military; and
3. build capacity within SAMHS so it can conduct research on other diseases of critical importance to military force preparedness. (SANDF 2006)

Participation in Phidisa clinical trials is voluntary. SAMHS expects that over a period of five years, about 50 000 soldiers and their dependants will have signed on to Phidisa. Three sites have been established in urban centres: Pretoria, Cape Town and Bloemfontein. Three other sites are located in rural areas: Phalaborwa, Mthatha and Matubatuba. These sites are equipped with the infrastructure to deliver HIV/AIDS support, care and treatment and to conduct clinical research. The project is divided into three phases or sets of activities. Phidisa I has been implemented as both a care and support programme and a study to better understand the links between HIV and risk-related co-infections in the SANDF. Phidisa II focuses more on ARV treatment and provides a treatment regimen to HIV-positive members and their dependants. Phidisa III, which has not yet been operationalised, will address issues such as African herbs and non-traditional medicines (Vuthela 2005).

The rationale behind Phidisa is directly related to questions about the impact of AIDS on the South African military. The Phidisa website notes, 'HIV has an impact on military preparedness. By identifying appropriate treatment for HIV infections, the project hopes to have a positive impact on military readiness. Among the treatments to be studied are anti-retroviral therapy, nutrition and traditional medicines.' (SANDF 2006) Project Phidisa aims to study the long-term treatment challenges within a South African context, which go beyond contemporary knowledge about the bio-medical efficacy of ARVs and are related to socio-economic, cultural and even political factors. For example, the project's researchers are assessing how local reliance on traditional medicine impacts on ARV adherence and efficacy. Poor roads, electricity and access to clean water also play a role in the administration of ARVs. These factors affect transportation to clinics, maintenance of adequate supplies of drugs and treatment of OIs in resource-poor environments.

Phidisa shared some of its findings at its yearly conference in Cape Town in August 2005. A study focusing on HIV/AIDS care and clinical research in rural areas provided some interesting information. The study involved 121 soldiers in Matubatuba and Mthatha participating in Phidisa and showed that socio-behavioural, clinical and operational research issues significantly impact on the administration of ARVs (Makatini et al. 2005). These issues encompassed a range of socio-economic, cultural, and even political factors, including:

- the importance of recognising strong belief systems;
- the need to effectively integrate traditional healers in HIV/AIDS care and support;

- the struggle to manage scarce resources in settings of extreme poverty;
- forecasting drug demand and assuring uninterrupted drug supply;
- managing space and time (HIV-positive participants in distant regions);
- planning and deploying a company; and
- creating peer-to-peer learning systems at clinic, district and country levels. (Makatini et al. 2005)

These issues illustrate several points. First, behaviour influenced by cultural beliefs remains central to the question of an adequate prevention and treatment response, even within a military setting. Second, social services and infrastructure are an important consideration for treating HIV/AIDS. Phidisa has taken steps to provide auxiliary, but essential services, such as nutritional support, allowances and transportation costs for its participants. Finally, according to a confidential source in March 2006, the SANDF is deeply concerned about ARV resistance. The programme has a strict process for participation in treatment. SANDF members and their families must demonstrate the capacity to comply with their medical regimens, but these steps require involvement from a wider social network going beyond the soldier and even his/her family.

Concluding remarks

The existing debate on human security is fundamentally about the nature of threats. The United Nations Development Programme's (UNDP) 1994 definition of human security drew attention to individuals and threats to their well-being. This definition of security widened the lens of security policy beyond traditional realist concerns for territorial integrity and the legitimate monopoly of force (see UNDP 1994; Chapter 1 in this volume). Human security, as a new framework, has sought to reinsert the well-being of people into governance (see Chapter 3 in this volume). It has been a tool, for example, to generate political will and financial resources to meet the needs of the most vulnerable people in Africa and elsewhere.

With varying degrees of usefulness, the human security framework has thus been applied to questions of vulnerability and is influencing governments in their response to HIV/AIDS in Africa. Human security, however, has not been widely applied to the traditional security actor of the military. Instead, traditional security actors, such as the UN Security Council, have sought to galvanise a response to the pandemic because of fears that militaries will crumble under the burden of AIDS (see Chapter 11 in this volume). However, the military, a pillar of state security, is the site for a nexus between human security-inspired policy and traditional security. First, the military's capacity or capability is linked to its human resources at individual and organisational levels. By affecting the health and well-being of its serving members, HIV/AIDS has the potential to deteriorate a military's capacity and capability. Second, HIV/AIDS is a disease driven by social behaviour, but rooted in a confluence of gendered social, economic and political factors (see Chapter 2 in this volume). Unlike other health burdens, such as injury in the field, HIV/AIDS requires comprehensive societal approaches, which fit neatly into a human security paradigm.

At the same time, the state's security is a porous assemblage of military, political, economic and social elements. Barry Buzan has written about defensive and offensive factors to a military's capacity to promote and protect security (1991, 66). According to Buzan, military concerns are part of a wider set of political, economic, socio-cultural and environmental fundamentals necessary for state security. Indeed, the defence and offensive capacity of a military to protect territorial integrity, sovereignty and stability are not isolated, but part of a wider spectrum of state functions and responsibilities. Here again, it is evident that what occurs politically, economically, environmentally and culturally interplays with military security. Thus human security *is* state security and vice versa. Indeed, just as they prioritise the procurement of military hardware, or the negotiation of collective security pacts with other states, security actors must fully embrace the value and meaning of what happens within a society.

In November 2007, the South African DoD organised an international conference on the impact of HIV and AIDS on combat readiness. The meeting explicitly encouraged discussion among HIV/AIDS medical experts from SAMHS, senior defence department officials and high-ranking officers from other branches of the SANDF.[6] As a beginning, the conference highlighted a shift toward co-operation and acknowledged the need to bring all of the DoD and the SANDF's other branches into a dialogue on the security dimensions of HIV/AIDS.

The SANDF's Masibambisane and Project Phidisa are complementary, just as prevention and treatment are mutually reinforcing. While Masibambisane does not offer ARV therapy, Phidisa does. The defence force faces several challenges, including how to:

- manage the costs of long-term HIV/AIDS treatment;
- transform the unequal gender relations that drive the epidemic;
- unravel the practical dilemmas related to long deployments of troops on peacekeeping missions;
- tackle the issue of retraining and finding new roles for HIV-positive troops who may no longer be able to carry out their duties;
- prevent the loss of high-level, specialised technical skills; and
- pre-empt a negative impact on its overall force strength. (Confidential sources, May 2005 and March 2006)[7]

These issues require further exploration in order to devise policy prescriptions (Barnett and Prins 2006, 8). However, these programmes, as discussed above, also address broader societal dimensions, since HIV/AIDS is inextricably part of broader social, cultural, political and economic realities, such as a lack of social infrastructure, social values and traditional beliefs. Today, security actors must address new issues, such as gender equality and psycho-social counselling, home-based care for the ill and how traditional medicine affects adherence to ARV treatment regimens.

HIV/AIDS is a wide-reaching societal phenomenon. The epidemic can affect military security because it impacts on the human resources of a defence force and because it is a threat to the whole of a society's well-being. Debating whether or not it is a human security or traditional threat is superfluous and understanding the response of militaries to HIV/AIDS from as broad a spectrum as possible is essential.

Notes

1. This chapter is based on research conducted by the Cape Town-based Centre for Conflict Resolution (CCR) in 2004 and 2005. The author is indebted to Dawn Alley, who carried out desk-based research on the SANDF and its HIV/AIDS management policies and practices on behalf of CCR.
2. South African policy-making and activist communities distinguish between Human Immunodeficiency Virus (HIV) – the virus – and Acquired Immunodeficiency Syndrome (AIDS), the condition that eventually ensues when HIV is left untreated. SAMHS and other government programmes therefore do not use 'HIV/AIDS', but 'HIV and AIDS' in their documents.
3. The current Surgeon-General is a former MK underground operative and was imprisoned on Robben Island before the end of apartheid. He led the MK military health team for integration into the NPKF (National Peacekeeping Force) and later the SANDF.

4. In May 2005, the author visited SAMHS personnel in Pretoria and met officers from several African countries who were participating in SAMHS training. The author has also interviewed HIV/AIDS programme heads from the Zimbabwe, Lesotho and Namibian defence forces who have attended SAMHS conferences and training.

5. *Phidisa* means 'to heal' in Setswana, one of South Africa's eleven official languages. In the early years of the project, the word '*phidisa*' was translated as 'make better/prolong life'.

6. The author was a participant at this conference and delivered a presentation on behalf of the CCR.

7. For a useful and practical guide on the impact of HIV/AIDS for the military sector, see HEARD 2005.

References

Adefalolu, A. 1999. 'HIV/AIDS as an Occupational Hazard to Soldiers: ECOMOG Experience'. Paper presented at the 3rd All Africa Congress of Armed Forces and Police Medical Services, Pretoria. Quoted in Alan Whiteside, Alex de Waal and Tsadkan Gebre-Tensae. 2006. 'AIDS, Security and the Military in Africa: A Sober Appraisal'. *African Affairs* 105(419): 201–18.

AU (African Union). 2004. *Human Security Report* and *Draft Text of the Common African Defence and Security Policy*, adopted at the AU Heads of State and Government Summit, Addis Ababa, Ethiopia, 7-9 July 2004.

AU (African Union) Peace and Security Council. 2002. *Protocol Relating to the Establishment of the Peace and Security Council of the African Union*. 1st Ordinary Session of the Assembly of the Heads of State. Available at http://www.africa-union.org/root/au/Documents/Treaties/Text/Protocol_peace%20and%20security.pdf, accessed 29 September 2006.

Barnett, Tony and Gwyn Prins. 2006. *HIV/AIDS and Security: Fact, Fiction, and Evidence: A Report to UNAIDS*. Geneva: UNAIDS; London: London School of Economics.

Berhe, Tadesse, Hagos Gemechu and Alex de Waal. 2005. 'War and HIV Prevalence: Evidence from Tigray, Ethiopia'. *African Security Review* 14(3): 107-14.

Buzan, Barry. 1991. *People, States and Fear: An Agenda for International Security Studies in the Post-Cold War Era*. Boulder: Lynne Rienner.

CCR (Centre for Conflict Resolution). 2005. 'HIV/AIDS and Human Security: An Agenda for Africa'. Available at http://ccrweb.ccr.uct.ac.za, accessed 16 April 2006.

———. 2006. 'HIV/AIDS and Southern Africa's Militaries'. Available at http://ccrweb.ccr.uct.ac.za, accessed 19 June 2006.

Cilliers, Jakkie and Mark Malan. 2005. 'Progress with the African Standby Force'. ISS Paper 107. Pretoria: Institute for Security Studies.

De Waal, Alex. 2006. *AIDS and Power: Why There Is No Political Crisis – Yet*. Cape Town: David Philip; London and New York: Zed Books.

DoD (Department of Defence). 2006. *Defence Bulletin* 18/06, 17 March.

———. 2007. 'The Impact of HIV and AIDS on Combat Readiness'. Conference programme 12–14 November, Pretoria.

DoH (Department of Health). 2005. *National HIV and Syphilis Antenatal Sero-Prevalence Survey South Africa 2004*. Pretoria: DoH.

Garret, Laurie. 2005. *HIV and National Security: Where Are the Links?* New York: Council on Foreign Relations.

Global Defence. 2003. 'Peacekeeping, Keeping Peace'. Available at http://www.global-defence.com/2003/sandef_03.htm, accessed 21 June 2006.

Govender, Pregs. 2007. *Love and Courage: A Story of Insubordination*. Johannesburg: Jacana.

HEARD (Health Economics and HIV/AIDS Research Division). 2005. 'The Military Sector: AIDS Brief for Sectoral Planners and Managers'. Durban: HEARD, University of KwaZulu-Natal. Available at http://www.heard.org.za/publications/AidsBriefs/sec/military.pdf, accessed 12 March 2006.

Hosken, Graeme. 2004. 'No AIDS Crisis in SANDF'. *The Mercury* 3 August.

JCIE (Japan Centre for International Exchange). 2006. *Report on Monitoring and Evaluation Mechanisms for the Projects Supported by the United Nations Trust Fund for Human Security in the Field of Health and HIV/AIDS*. New York: JCIE.

Lekota, Mosiuoa (Minister of Defence). 2003. Speech on the occasion of the official launch of Project Phidisa. Available at http://www.health-e.org.za, accessed 1 December 2003.

Le Roux, Len. 2005. 'The Post-Apartheid South African Military: Transforming with the Nation'. In *Evolutions and Revolutions: A Contemporary History of Militaries in Southern Africa*, ed. Martin Rupiya, 235–66. Pretoria: Institute for Security Studies.

Le Roux, Len and Henri Boshoff. 2005. 'The State of the Military'. In *The State of the Nation 2004–2005*, ed. John Daniel, Roger Southall and Jessica Lutchman, 177–200. Cape Town: Human Sciences Research Council Press.

Makatini, Zinhle, Jorge Tavel, Japie Croukamp, Sbongiseni Dhlomo, Thandeka Khanyile, Sam Beja, Tokelo Madisha, Gugu Natchamba and Anita Lessing. 2005. *Challenges of Providing HIV/AIDS Care and Performing Clinical Research in Rural Settings: Lessons for South Africa's National Roll-Out Program*. Pretoria: SANDF; Washington, DC: National Institute for Health, Henry Jackson, Clindev.

Michaels, Jeremy. 2004. 'What Future Awaits HIV-Positive Soldiers?' *The Star* 18 August.

Nattrass, Nicoli. 2002. 'AIDS and Human Security in Southern Africa'. CSSR Working Paper No. 18. Cape Town: Centre for Social Science Research.

Rupiya, Martin (ed.). 2005. *Evolutions and Revolutions: A Contemporary History of Militaries in Southern Africa*. Pretoria: Institute for Security Studies.

———. 2006. *The Enemy Within: Southern African Militaries' Quarter-Century Battle with HIV/AIDS*. Pretoria: Institute for Security Studies.

SAMHS (South African Military Health Services). n.d. 'Core Business'. Available at http://www.mhs.mil.za/corebusiness/corebusiness.htm, accessed 20 June 2006.

———. 2005. *The Comprehensive Plan for the Holistic Management of HIV and AIDS in the Department of Defence: 2005–2010*. Pretoria: SAMHS.

———. 2005–06. 'Masibambisane'. Available at http://www.mhs.mil.za/masi/index.htm, accessed 23 June 2006.

SAMHS News. 2006. 'Well Done SAMHS!' Available at http://www.mhs.mil.za/news/news2006/may/24may_address.htm, accessed 23 June 2006.

SANDF (South African National Defence Force). 1998. *South African Defence Review*. Pretoria: DoD.

———. 2006. 'Phidisa: "Make Better, Prolong Life"'. Available at http://www.phidisa.org/about.html, accessed 19 June 2006.

UNAIDS (Joint United Nations Programme for HIV/AIDS). 1998. *AIDS and the Military*. New York and Geneva: UNAIDS. Also cited in remarks made by the UNAIDS Executive Director, Dr Peter Piot, 22 September 2003, at UN General Assembly High-Level Meeting on HIV/AIDS, New York.

———. 2006. 'Report on the Global AIDS Epidemic'. UNAIDS/06.20E.

UNAIDS (Joint United Nations Programme for HIV/AIDS) and WHO (World Health Organisation). 2004. 'AIDS Epidemic Update'. UNAIDS/04.E.

———. 2005. 'AIDS Epidemic Update Report'. Geneva and New York: UNAIDS/WHO.

UN Department of Peacekeeping Operations. n.d. 'Factsheet'. Available at http://www.un.org/Depts/dpko/factsheet.pdf, accessed 24 September 2006 and descriptions of current peacekeeping operations, available at http://www.un.org/Depts/dpko/dpko/, accessed 24 September 2006.

UNDP (United Nations Development Programme). 1994. *New Dimensions of Human Security*. Human Development Report. Available at http://www.hdr.undp.org/reports/global/ 1994/en/, accessed 2 May 2007.

Vuthela, Nomonde. 2005. 'The Many Faces of Phidisa'. *SA Soldier*, December: 26. Pretoria.

10

The Development Agenda and HIV/AIDS

———— • ————

Alan Whiteside

Introduction

The HIV/AIDS epidemic was first recognised in 1981, more than 28 years ago, among gay men in the United States. Since the first cases were identified, at least 20 million people have died of the disease and some 33 million have been infected. At the end of 2007, the Joint United Nations Programme on HIV/AIDS (UNAIDS) released new estimates of the number of infected people, which caused some consternation, as there was a significant reduction in the global numbers. In 2006 it had been estimated that there were 39.5 million people living with the virus. The 2007 report reduced this number by 6.3 million, to 33.2 million (UNAIDS and WHO 2007).

An important feature of the epidemic is that HIV is not spread (or spreading) uniformly around the world; the bulk of infections are in Africa. Yet even in this case, some regions on the continent are much more affected than others. Sub-Saharan Africa is home to two-thirds of global infections. UNAIDS estimated that 32 per cent of the world's HIV infections and 34 per cent of AIDS deaths globally were in southern African countries (UNAIDS and WHO 2007, 9). By contrast, HIV prevalence remained static at low levels in most of West Africa and had fallen in East Africa (2007, 6).

The decline in infection rates means that our understanding of the epidemic, its spread and its effects, needs to be nuanced. Furthermore, we need to appreciate why and where the numbers have been reduced. Prevalence figures are compiled primarily from national data and are subject to review by the UNAIDS Reference Group on Estimates, Modelling and Projections, based at the Imperial College in London. UNAIDS and the World Health Organisation (WHO) say the decline in infection rates is due to better surveillance and modelling. In the past, data relied on surveys of pregnant women (usually) in state antenatal clinics. Over the last five years, there have been demographic and health surveys (DHSs) in many countries, particularly in Africa. These provide population-based data across countries of men and women in rural and urban areas.

The greatest part of the 6.3 million global decline in prevalence figures in 2007 came from a radical downward revision of the data from India. In 2006, it was estimated that there were 5.2 million infections in India. The latest data suggest that there are about 2.5 million infections (UNAIDS and WHO 2007, 21). UNAIDS identifies other countries, such as Angola, India, Kenya, Nigeria, Mozambique and Zimbabwe, which also contributed significantly to the decline in global infection rates (2007, 9). But there is a need for caution, even with the improved data and methodology. Experience and knowledge of what is occurring suggests that data from Nigeria and Zimbabwe are probably not reliable. In Nigeria data reported by UNAIDS in 2006 came from surveys conducted at only 10 urban and 70 rural sites in 2001. There was no indication in 2007 that there are better or updated figures for Nigeria. In Zimbabwe it is hard to believe that reliable HIV data are being collected, in the context of an overstretched health system and a collapsing economy. These questions of data are important. Figures are needed to show the impact of prevention efforts and to plan for increasing demands placed on healthcare and other social services.

The 2007 data show that the burden of AIDS as a development issue will primarily impact most on East and southern Africa. The potential links between AIDS and development and conversely, between development and the spread of HIV, were recognised early in the epidemic by a small number of scholars and development practitioners. Early work by economists, for example, suggested that increasing numbers of AIDS cases and deaths would cause economic growth to slow. It was argued that projects that facilitated the movement of people, particularly of young single men (such as construction of dams and roads) could increase HIV transmission. Sadly, little notice was taken of these warnings (see, for example, Cohen 1992; Bloom and Lyons 1993; Cross and Whiteside 1993).

Development is a national and international goal. This chapter is an assessment of the HIV/AIDS and development nexus in the light of the growing impact of the pandemic. It begins by setting out why HIV/AIDS is such a unique disease and examines the concept of long-wave events. It then explores how development has been defined nationally and internationally and how HIV/AIDS can influence development, using as an example one particular development goal: reducing child mortality. It also assesses some of the major international development initiatives of 2005. Finally it describes how development influences the spread of HIV.

HIV/AIDS as a development issue

The disease-development nexus is not a new phenomenon. Perhaps the most dramatic recorded example of how disease can impact on societies is the effect of European diseases on the indigenous peoples of the Americas. Outbreaks began with the arrival of Christopher Columbus in 1492, followed by the march of Spanish conquistadores into South and Central America and the settlement of North America by the British and French. The early American epidemics were overwhelming. The population of central Mexico – the Aztec realm – fell from an estimated 25.2 million people in 1518 to about 700 000 in 1623, a 97 per cent decline in little over a century (Mann 2005). What this meant for society and development in these areas has not been explored (which is unfortunate, as such analyses could be instructive for those trying to understand today's HIV/AIDS epidemic).

The current AIDS epidemic began spreading in the 1970s (Iliffe 2006, 10). The history of the spread of HIV in the United States has been well documented by Randy Shilts (1988) and in Africa by John Iliffe (2006). It is likely that the reason HIV took hold in the 1970s and spread so rapidly was, at least in part, the result of 'development'. Increased mobility allowed the virus to move from city to city and from continent to continent. Expanding transport infrastructure meant that many communities were easily reachable and the virus could be transmitted across countries and borders in a few days. Linked to this was the rapid urbanisation of the 1970s and 1980s, especially in Africa: 'More immediately, population growth drove Africa's massive late-twentieth-century urbanisation – at about 5 per cent per year during the 1980s – which created cities like Kinshasa and Abidjan, where networks of partner exchange were wide enough to raise HIV to epidemic levels' (Iliffe 2006, 60). However, it was not only due to increased mobility that HIV/AIDS was able to take hold in Africa. The nature of 'development' in Africa was highly inequitable both in terms of material wealth and gender relations (Barnett and Whiteside 2006).

There are three biological features of HIV that make it unique with regard to development. First, it is a retrovirus. It has ribonucleic acid (RNA) as its genetic material and it invades cells of the human immune system in order to reproduce.

Within these cells, it produces more virus particles by converting viral RNA into deoxyribonucleic acid (DNA) and then making RNA copies. The switch from RNA to DNA and back to RNA makes combating HIV complex, as it results in small errors leading to the mutation of the virus. Thus it is difficult to treat as it can develop resistance. There are drugs available, but they are expensive, must be taken for the life of the patient and do not cure, but only suppress the virus.

Second, HIV is a lentivirus: a slow-acting virus. There is a long period, on average ten years, between infection and illness. During this period, the disease can be transmitted, but people generally do not know they are infected. This makes the disease and its impacts a 'long-wave event'.

Third, while the virus is present in all body fluids of infected persons, the greatest concentrations are in blood, semen and vaginal secretions. This has implications for how it is transmitted and who is infected. Exposure to blood or blood products carries the maximum risk, hence the concern around blood safety and hygiene in healthcare settings. It is also why there are high levels of transmission among injecting drug users who use non-sterile injecting equipment. However, the most common mode of transmission is sexual intercourse: 75–85 per cent of HIV-positive people in the world are infected this way. Heterosexual transmission and mother-to-child transmission (MTCT) in the intrauterine period, during childbirth and through breastfeeding are the most prevailing routes of HIV infection in Africa.

As HIV is predominantly sexually transmitted, there is a very specific age distribution of infections. Most infections are among adults aged 20–45. Where the epidemic is heterosexually driven, more women are infected and at a younger age than men. Figure 10.1 shows the gender and age distribution of infections in South Africa in 2005 and is typical of heterosexually transmitted epidemics across Africa. As shown in this graph, infection rates are considerably higher among young women between the ages of 15 and 30 and peak in the 25–29 age group. Infection levels among men peak in their thirties.

The long-term implications of HIV/AIDS

HIV/AIDS is a long-wave event. Tony Barnett has suggested that the defining qualities of long-wave events are:

- they last decades and perhaps centuries;
- their effects are seen before their longer-run significance, weight or cause are appreciated; and

- 'emergency' reactions taken for the ostensible good can have long-term consequences that *exacerbate* the problem. (Barnett 2006, 297–313, especially 303; Barnett and Prins 2006)

HIV/AIDS fits this bill. At an individual level, the period from infection to illness and then death may be more than ten years. At a population level, epidemiologists suggest that it might take 100 years or more for the epidemic to run its course, since the impacts of the epidemic take generations to work through the population. For example, in Rakai province in Uganda, children who were orphaned in the first wave of the epidemic are leaving a new generation of orphans. In South Africa, older women have traditionally been at the core of many families. The median age at which a woman becomes a grandmother is 40 (Chazan 2006). In twenty years' time, however, a large cohort of grandmothers will be missing because they are dying.

The increased mortality among young women in South Africa is illustrated by Figure 10.2. This chart shows the actual number of recorded deaths, yearly and by age cohort from 1997 to 2004. Most of those dying in 2004 were infected in the early years of the epidemic, between 1992 and 1997, when HIV prevalence among pregnant women attending antenatal clinics rose from just over 2 per cent to about 16 per cent. By 2004, HIV prevalence was close to 30 per cent.

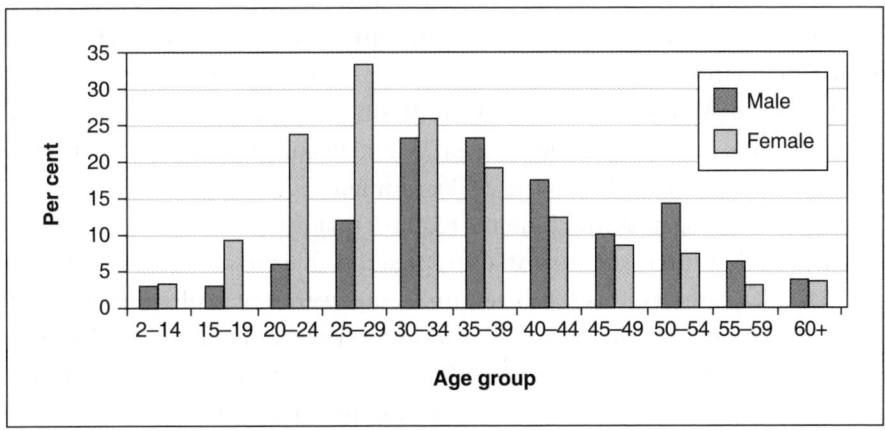

Figure 10.1 HIV prevalence by sex and age, South Africa, 2005.

Source: Shisana et al. 2005

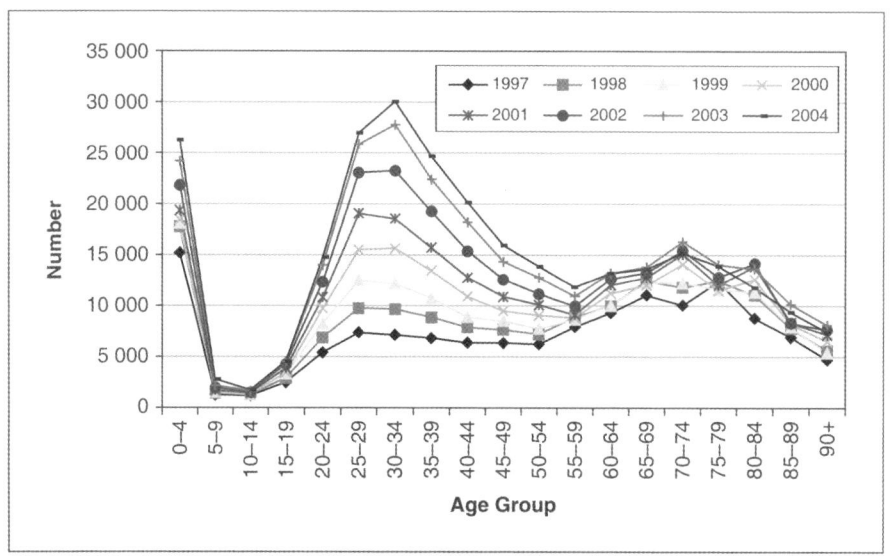

Figure 10.2 Female mortality in South Africa, 1997–2004.

Source: Stats SA 2006

It is difficult for decision-makers and planners to understand the long-term implications of HIV/AIDS. It takes time before there are sufficient deaths for the disease to be visible. Even then, mortality is spread across a country and given the stigma associated with the virus, AIDS deaths often remain invisible. This makes it difficult to convince policy-makers of the need to mount responses early in the epidemic, although in South Africa this common dynamic has been exacerbated by the government's own unique blend of AIDS denialism, which has further retarded its response to the epidemic (Fourie 2006; Gumede 2005).

Effective action against the epidemic requires that people believe in the existence of the disease, that it has the potential to spread in their society and that it poses a threat. An adequate response also requires empowerment. All southern African leaders are aware of the threat HIV/AIDS poses to their populations. What they do not seem to understand is the adverse effects it will have on development, nor do they seem to appreciate that responding to the disease requires long-term actions. However, African leaders are not alone; large parts of the global community also choose to ignore the epidemic and its development implications.

What is development?

Human nature demands that people strive to improve their lives. For some, this means accumulating material possessions; for others, intellectual advancement and for many, that the world be a better place for their children. Economic development is generally viewed as a sustained increase in living standards, which includes rising incomes, better health and improved education and the opportunity for people to achieve their potential.

The goal of development is both national and global. All nations expect to make progress. In the developed world, this ambition is set out in political manifestos. In the developing world, goals are most often articulated through national development plans or poverty reduction strategy programmes. Botswana's ninth National Development Plan (2003–04 to 2008–09), for example, has as its theme 'Sustainable and Diversified Development through Competitiveness in Global Markets'. Presenting the Plan in parliament, Baledzi Gaolathe, Minister of Finance and Development Planning, noted that the plan 'aims at building the pillars of Vision 2016, namely, an educated and informed nation; a prosperous, productive and innovative nation; a compassionate, just and caring nation; a safe and secure nation; an open, democratic and accountable nation; a moral and tolerant nation; and a united and proud nation' (Gaolathe 2002). Delivering development is a political goal. People are more likely to vote for a party or a politician promising a better future for themselves and their children. Setting national goals is usually not contentious and the targets are generally bland. There is not much variation between parties or even countries.

The idea of development is also prominent at the international level. There are agencies with the specific task of achieving development. Multilateral agencies include, for example, the United Nations Development Programme (UNDP) and the World Bank. Most rich countries have their own bilateral programmes, such as the Swedish International Development Agency (SIDA) and the United Kingdom's Department for International Development (DfID).

There has been one initiative to set global targets: the Millennium Development Goals (MDGs), which were adopted in 2000 by the United Nations (UN) General Assembly (UN General Assembly 2000, 1; UN 2000). The second paragraph of the General Assembly's resolution on the MDGs states: 'we have a collective responsibility to uphold the principles of human dignity, equality and equity at the global level.

As leaders we have a duty therefore to all the world's people, especially the most vulnerable' (UN 2007). There are eight MDGs and eighteen targets. The first seven goals relate to life conditions in the resource-poor world. Goal 8 and targets 12–18 are about developing a global partnership for development (see below). Goals 4–6 relate to health, specifically maternal mortality, child mortality and disease. The two diseases specifically named are HIV/AIDS and malaria. In setting the MDGs, the impact of HIV/AIDS on development was largely ignored, as the discussion on the child mortality goal illustrates. Perhaps there was some excuse for this at the end of the 1990s, when global targets were being established. However, as this chapter shows, HIV/AIDS and its complexity continue to be ignored.

The Millennium Development Goals

Goal 1: Eradicate extreme poverty and hunger
Target 1. Halve, between 1990 and 2015, the proportion of people whose income is less than US$1 a day.
Target 2. Halve, between 1990 and 2015, the proportion of people who suffer from hunger.

Goal 2: Achieve universal primary education
Target 3. Ensure that, by 2015, children everywhere, boys and girls alike, will be able to complete a full course of primary schooling.

Goal 3: Promote gender equality and empower women
Target 4. Eliminate gender disparities in primary and secondary education, preferably by 2005, and in all levels of education by no later than 2015.

Goal 4: Reduce child mortality
Target 5. Reduce by two-thirds, between 1990 and 2015, the under-five mortality rate.

Goal 5: Improve maternal health
Target 6. Reduce by three-quarters, between 1990 and 2015, the maternal mortality ratio.

Goal 6: Combat HIV/AIDS, malaria and other diseases
Target 7. Have halted by 2015 and begun to reverse the spread of HIV/AIDS.

Target 8.   Have halted by 2015 and begun to reverse the incidence of malaria and
other major diseases.

Goal 7: Ensure environmental sustainability
Target 9.   Integrate the principles of sustainable development into country policies
and programs and reverse the loss of environmental resources.
Target 10. Halve, by 2015, the proportion of people without sustainable access to safe
drinking water and basic sanitation.
Target 11. Have achieved by 2020 a significant improvement in the lives of at least
100 million slum dwellers.

Goal 8: Develop a global partnership for development
Target 12. Develop an open trading and financial system that is rule-based, predictable,
and non-discriminatory.
Target 13. Address the least developed countries' special needs through tariff- and
quota-free access for their exports, enhanced debt relief, cancellation of
bilateral debt, and more generous official development assistance for
countries committed to poverty reduction.
Target 14. Address the special needs of landlocked and small island developing states.
Target 15. Deal comprehensively with developing countries' debt problems through
national and international measures to make debt sustainable in the long
term.
Target 16. In co-operation with the developing countries, develop decent and productive
work for youth.
Target 17. In co-operation with pharmaceutical companies, provide access to affordable
essential drugs in developing countries.
Target 18. In co-operation with the private sector, make available the benefits of new
technologies – especially information and communications technologies.
(UN 2000; UN General Assembly 2000)

Disease, death and development

The impact of HIV/AIDS stems from increased illness and death. The effects range
from slower macro-economic growth to desperate poverty among those who have
fallen ill and those who are caring for orphans and the sick. Much has already been
written about these subjects. This chapter focuses on only one issue: the demographic

impact of AIDS and specifically its impact on the fourth MDG of reducing child mortality.

Demography examines populations and dynamics. It is concerned with the numbers and structure of populations. Demographers measure and predict population size and growth rates; structure by gender and age and key indicators such as birth, death and fertility rates, life expectancy, and infant and child mortality.

There are three major problems that need to be appreciated when assessing demographic indicators. First, these indicators address events, rather than processes. HIV/AIDS is a process: a person becomes ill, does not grow as much food, or is unable to work, which might, for example, result in his/her family having less income and being unable to afford to send children to school. The demographer records a death, its effect on household composition and dependency ratios, but not the impact of the events leading up to the death or those flowing from it. Second, demographic indicators focus on nations, provinces or areas. The impact of the disease may be concentrated among specific groups and in households. Some people may be pushed into desperate poverty, while others cope, or even improve their status. The third problem is that data reflect the past. Censuses epitomise this, since they are carried out every ten years. This means we are looking retroactively at an event that is unfolding in the present and will extend and amplify in the future.

The impact on female mortality

AIDS increases mortality in adult age groups that would otherwise typically have the lowest mortality rates. In Rakai, Uganda, a team of researchers followed a cohort of 19 983 adults aged 15–59 at ten-monthly intervals over four surveys in the 1990s. HIV prevalence in this cohort was 16.1 per cent. The mortality rate among HIV-positive people in the cohort was 132.6 per 1 000 person years, while in HIV-negative people, it was only 6.7 (Sewankambo et al. 2000, 391–400). HIV-positive people were nineteen times more likely to die than their uninfected peers.

South Africa's system of vital registration shows mortality and trends. This is shown for women in Figure 10.2. Deaths among women have increased since 1997. Notably, however, in 1997, the greatest numbers of deaths were among women in their late seventies. By 2004, death rates were highest among women in their thirties, with the number of deaths in this age group having increased nearly six-fold over the eight-year period (Stats SA 2006).

The impact on child mortality

Child mortality rates increase because children born to infected mothers may be infected and even if these children are uninfected themselves, they are more likely to die if they lose their mothers. In the absence of appropriate interventions, a child born to an HIV-positive mother has about a 30 per cent chance of being infected. The likelihood of transmission prior to or during birth can be reduced by two-thirds by administering a single dose of the antiretroviral (ARV) drug, Nevirapine to the mother. MTCT can also be reduced much further by a combination of ARVs over several weeks. Infected infants are likely to die young. The death of a mother (from any cause) increases the chance of a child dying three-fold in the year before the mother's death and five times in the year after her death. This increased mortality is not influenced by what the mother died of, but HIV-infected mothers are, of course, more likely to die (Newell, Brahmbhatt and Ghys 2004).

There are a number of sources for indicators of child mortality shifts in South Africa. Statistics South Africa (Stats SA) and other organisations report a decrease in infant mortality since 2001, the year that the South African government first began rolling out its treatment programme for preventing MTCT of HIV (for more on the history of government distribution of ARVs in South Africa, see Chapter 3 in this volume). The South African Presidency's mid-term review of development indicators in 2007 cited estimates on the rates of children who died within the first year of birth (infant mortality). The report shows that in 2001, infant mortality was at 28 per 1 000 live births. However, infant mortality stood at 38.1 per 1 000 live births in 2004 and Department of Health (DoH) statistics report about 43 infant deaths for every 1 000 live births (Office of the Presidency of South Africa 2007).

The cumulative toll

The UN Population Division is the leading source of international population data. In 2003, the agency produced a sobering report looking at the impact of HIV/AIDS. Table 10.1, developed from the report, shows the data for life expectancy and child mortality for five-year intervals from 1995–2000 to 2020–25. In the absence of the epidemic, improvements in both indicators were expected. The effects of HIV/AIDS are particularly marked in higher prevalence countries. While HIV/AIDS reduces life expectancy in all of the 53 countries studied, in the 7 countries with HIV prevalence of over 20 per cent, life expectancy will decline by over 40 per cent and fall as low as 37.6 years by 2025. The epidemic will also reverse the gains in child

Table 10.1 Estimated and projected impact of HIV/AIDS on life expectancy and child mortality indicators.

Indicator	53 countries where HIV/AIDS impact was included in 2002 UN estimates			7 countries with prevalence > than 20 per cent		
	1995–2000	2010–15	2020–25	1995–2000	2010–15	2020–25
Life expectancy at birth (years)						
Without AIDS	63.9	68.4	70.8	62.3	67.0	69.6
With AIDS	62.4	64.2	65.9	50.2	37.6	41.0
Percentage difference	2.4	6.1	6.9	19.3	43.9	41.1
Child mortality rate (per 1 000)						
Without AIDS	93.9	68.8	56.1	80.2	56.9	44.8
With AIDS	98.8	75.8	62.3	108.8	100.2	84.3
Percentage difference	5.3	10.0	11.1	35.7	76.2	88.4

Source: UN Secretariat 2003, 185

mortality achieved over the last 50 years, with levels of mortality expected to increase by an astounding 88 per cent between 2020 and 2025 (UN Secretariat 2003).

The international response

HIV/AIDS has been high on the international agenda since 2000, when it was first mooted as a security issue (see Chapter 11 in this volume). In January 2000, in a statement to the UN Security Council, the US Vice-President Al Gore warned that HIV/AIDS posed a threat to institutions that were the guardians of nations. Calling for a new definition of security, he cautioned that HIV/AIDS was weakening workforces and could affect economic and military power. HIV/AIDS was in effect, a new type of security issue: 'this meeting demands of us that we see security through a new and wider prism, and forever after, think about it according to a new, more expansive definition' (cited in Behrman 2004, 164).

In July 2000, the UN Security Council passed Resolution 1 308, which stated that if left unaddressed, the HIV/AIDS pandemic would constitute a risk to peace and security (UNSC 2000). In June 2001, the UN General Assembly held a Special Session on HIV/AIDS (UNGASS), which called for an urgent and sustained response. Subsequent to this there were three new major initiatives specific to HIV/AIDS. The

UN Secretary-General Kofi Annan called for spending on HIV/AIDS to be increased ten-fold in developing countries. In 2001, the establishment of the Global Fund to Fight AIDS, Tuberculosis and Malaria (GFATM) was announced. Annan wanted US$10 billion as seed money for the fund and the global response to HIV/AIDS, but initially only US$1.6 billion was raised. A second scheme, the US$15 billion US Presidential Emergency Programme for AIDS Relief (PEPFAR), provided funding to fifteen developing countries, mainly in sub-Saharan Africa. Finally, the World Health Organisation's (WHO) new director-general, Lee Jong-Wook, named HIV/AIDS as his top priority in his first speech, declaring that the failure to deliver treatment was a global public health emergency. On 1 December 2003 (World AIDS Day), he announced, with UNAIDS, a new '3-by-5' plan, which aimed to treat three million people in poor countries by the end of 2005.

This chapter does not take issue with these specific HIV/AIDS initiatives, but rather looks at the role of the international community as it articulated efforts to address development and HIV/AIDS in 2005 through various international forums and reports. It focuses on the Africa Commission, the mid-term reporting on the MDGs and the subsequent World Summit.

The Africa Commission

The Africa Commission was established by British Prime Minister Tony Blair in 2004 and submitted its report in early 2005. The Commission's report proposed a 'coherent package' for Africa to address the interrelated problems of under-development, which include poor governance, a lack of growth, environmental degradation, adverse terms of trade and debt. It argued that these challenges had to be met through a new kind of partnership and development approach, which would need to be based on mutual respect and solidarity, as well as the need for an analysis of policies that had been effective (Africa Commission 2005).

The Commission suggested that as part of the solution, more money was needed in foreign assistance: an additional US$25 billion per year in aid by 2010, and a further US$25 billion per year by 2015. A review of the report shows that the actions envisaged included:

- investment in African capacity;
- supporting accountable budgetary processes and anti-corruption measures;
- supporting conflict management structures and processes;

- funding educational and healthcare services;
- supporting economic growth and poverty reduction strategies; and
- the promotion of more and fairer trade.

The Commission's report has just one subsection devoted to HIV/AIDS in the chapter 'Leaving No-One out: Investing in People'. The 'Growing for Growth and Poverty Reduction' chapter identifies the economic impact of HIV/AIDS as a key challenge: 'Top priority must be given to scaling up services needed to deal with the catastrophe of HIV and AIDS . . . But this must be done through existing systems, rather than parallel new ones. Governments should also be supported to protect orphans and vulnerable children and other groups who would otherwise be left out of the growth story.' (Africa Commission 2005)

The recommendations of the Commission's report are unexceptional and the only innovative idea is that the HIV and AIDS response should be mainstreamed and UNAIDS should develop accreditation systems for HIV and AIDS competency among governments, international agencies and the private sector. Other suggestions are predictable: the international community should reach global agreement to harmonise the incongruent and unco-ordinated response to the pandemic and donors should increase their contribution to US$10 billion, along the same lines as targets set by UNGASS.

The UN Millennium Goal reporting and the World Summit in 2005

The release of the Millennium Development Report in 2005 was the most comprehensive review of progress towards the MDGs (UN Statistics Division 2005). In his foreword to the report, Kofi Annan highlighted the risk that many of the world's developing countries would not meet a number of goals. Overall, the data are not encouraging, especially for the poorest countries, many of whom will not meet the targets and some of whom are already falling behind significantly. As a British Broadcasting Corporation (BBC) report on 12 September 2005 noted, 'sub-Saharan Africa appears to be moving backwards rather than forwards' (Black 2005).

Rates of extreme poverty declined in Asia, but in sub-Saharan Africa millions more fell deeply into poverty. While 30 countries have reduced hunger by at least 25 per cent during the past decade, in sub-Saharan Africa the number of malnourished children increased, partly as a result of conflicts, population growth and declining agricultural productivity (UN Statistics Division 2005). The report also shows the toll that HIV/AIDS is taking on child mortality. Countries afflicted by HIV/AIDS, especially in southern Africa, have seen increases in deaths among the under-fives. At current rates, it is estimated that the reduction in child mortality by 2015 will be about 15 per cent, as opposed to the two-thirds target set out in the MDGs.

Goal 6 of the MDGs aimed specifically to combat HIV/AIDS and malaria. However, these pandemics – and tuberculosis (TB) – remain the primary causes of premature death in the poorest countries of the world. Specifically on HIV/AIDS, the report attributes insufficient progress in tackling the epidemic to 'inadequate resources and a lack of political leadership . . . especially where HIV has established footholds among marginalised and stigmatised groups' (UN Statistics Division 2005, 6).

The overview of the MDGs and Kofi Annan's report, *In Larger Freedom: Towards Development, Security, and Human Rights for All,* identified a broad and varied list of reasons for the shortfalls in progress (UN Statistics Division 2005; UN 2005). The first reason is governance failures, when governments do not uphold the rule of law, human rights norms and do not create suitable economic policy, or make appropriate public investments. The second is the poverty trap, where countries are too poor to help themselves. The third is the existence of pockets of poverty that result in lagging regions or groups. Finally, there are areas of specific policy neglect where objectives were not met, largely due to ignorance on the part of policy-makers (UN 2005). HIV/AIDS warrants barely a mention in many economic, agricultural or investment policy documents, for example, and yet it is a cross-cutting issue that will affect developmental outcomes in the long term. Indeed, current data show that in 2015, when the MDGs are due, mortality and orphaning rates will still be rising in many countries.

The MDGs were discussed by 150 heads of state in New York at the World Summit held between 14 and 16 September 2005. The World Summit reiterated commitment to the promises made at the G8 Gleneagles summit in July 2005, adding a strong commitment to providing immediate support for 'quick impact' initiatives to support anti-malaria efforts, education and healthcare. Developed countries pledged an additional US$50 billion a year to fight poverty and reaffirmed their intention to deal with Africa's special needs. Leaders also resolved to put in place a lasting solution to the external debt burden of African countries (UN General Assembly 2005b).

The outcome document primarily confirmed commitments to broad principles and to working towards the achievement of established goals, rather than setting out precise objectives and timeframes. The adoption of a bold national development strategy by 2006 for each developing country with extreme poverty was approved in full. However, although promises by developed countries to achieve the 0.7 per cent target for official development assistance were welcomed, no pressure or deadlines were placed on them to reach this target (UN General Assembly 2005a, 2005b; UN News Service 2005).

The international responses summarised

This review of the events of 2005 shows how HIV is simply not on the global development agenda. Indeed, it is clear that the increased mortality and consequences for economies and society at large are not being considered. On the one hand, the UN Population Division shows greatly increased child mortality; on the other hand, the MDG assessment ignores this in reviewing the goals. There is simply not an appreciation of the nature of the disease and its impact, or any real understanding of the idea of long-wave events.

The role of development in the spread of HIV

In order for a person to become infected with HIV, they must be exposed to the virus, which will depend on their behaviour. Key drivers of HIV transmission are the age of sexual debut, sexual practices, number of partners, frequency of partner exchange, concurrency of partners and sexual mixing patterns. The younger a woman is when she begins having sex, the greater her risk of infection (see Chapter 2 in this volume). Globally, data suggest females have sex earlier than men and girls often feel pressured, or are forced into sex. In a recent national survey of young South Africans between the ages of 15 and 24, 28 per cent of females and 16 per cent of males indicated that they either 'did not want' or 'really did not want' their first sexual experience (Reproductive Health Research Unit 2004).

The question of sexual practices is one that receives more press and speculation than is deserved, although it is the area about which we know least. With regard to HIV transmission, the number of sexual partners is less important than the frequency of partner exchange – whether or not the partners are concurrent – and sexual mixing patterns. This has been confirmed by a range of DHSs across the world. Concurrency, where people have more than one partner and the relationships overlap for weeks, months, or years, is critical. Mathematical models comparing populations with serial monogamy and long-term concurrency showed that in the latter, HIV transmission would be much more rapid and the epidemic ten times greater. As Daniel Halperin and Helen Epstein note:

> The effect of such concurrency on the spread of HIV is exacerbated by the fact that viral load, and thus infectivity, is much higher during the initial weeks or months after infection. Therefore, as soon as one person in a network of concurrent relationships contracts HIV, everyone else in the network is placed at risk. By contrast, serial monogamy traps the virus within a single relationship for months or years. (2004, 5)

Mixing patterns are also important. These make it possible for an infection to be carried from one part of a country to another, across national borders, or to be introduced into previously closed circles.

When HIV was first identified, there was much emphasis on commercial sex as a medium of transmission. When the epidemic is beginning in any particular population, this concern is correct, as sex workers may be so-called 'core transmitters'. A modelling exercise by the World Bank showed that if the proportion of sex workers consistently using condoms in Nairobi increased from 10–80 per cent, 10 200 new infections would be prevented per year, although increasing condom use by the same amount among clients would have minimal impact (World Bank 1997). In Thailand, the early epidemic was spread by sex workers, but the '100 per cent Condom Campaign' was effective in bringing it under control. However, by the time the epidemic is established, as was the case across southern Africa, focusing on commercial sex alone is not sufficient. All sexual behaviours that might put people at risk need to be considered, including transactional and survival sex (Whiteside 2008). The relative power of the partners and ability to insist on condom use are also crucial factors (see Chapter 2 in this volume.)

Behaviours do not take place in isolation; they result from the environment in which people live and operate. The type of development experienced and how it plays out will be important in determining these behaviours. In South Africa, the early development of mines and industry required labour and thus influenced social relations in all their dimensions (see Chapter 2 in this volume.) Colonial and apartheid rule meant that black labour was less educated and exploited. Foreign migrant miners were drawn from Malawi, Lesotho, Botswana, Swaziland,

Mozambique and Namibia, while apartheid meant that many black South Africans were classified as migrants, effectively foreigners in their own country. The effects of this dislocation and disempowerment have been well documented by Catherine Campbell for the mining area of Carltonville near Johannesburg (2003). The confluence of the erosion of families through migrant labour, new sexual networks and disempowerment contributed to the transmission of HIV.

The relationship between HIV/AIDS and poverty is complex at the international, continental and individual level. There is no generalised epidemic in any of the Organisation for Economic Co-operation and Development (OECD) countries. The highest levels in Europe and North America are in Spain and the United States, where adult prevalence is 0.6 per cent. There are poor countries where HIV has not spread. On the African continent, Senegal is held up as an example. However, there are relatively wealthy developing countries where prevalence is very high. The two prime examples are Botswana and South Africa. Certain kinds of development alone, such as improving gross domestic product (GDP) per capita, will not necessarily prevent HIV spreading.

Initially in developing countries, being HIV-positive seemed to correlate with having higher incomes, especially among men. Men with higher incomes were more likely to have multiple partners, whether they purchased sex, or simply had more girlfriends. They could afford the partners and had more opportunity to find them. It was believed that, over time, the disease would be increasingly located among poorer people. However, data from demographic and health surveys and other longitudinal studies show that the picture is opaque. The issue is not simply how well off a person is, but rather about the structure of the society they live in and their relative well-being. Development is not neutral. Issues of equity and gender are crucial and this is beginning to be explored (Barnett and Whiteside 2006; De Waal 2006).

Conclusion

When the history of the first 50 years of the epidemic is written, it is likely that 2005 will mark the year when the disease got the most attention and greatest resources (relative to need). In fact, 2005 will probably mark the highest level of political mobilisation to address the disease in Africa. Yet, despite the rhetoric, understanding HIV/AIDS, how it will drive (under)development and how the type of development will affect the size and scale of the problem, have not yet been fully explored.

What is still lacking is an understanding of HIV/AIDS as a long-wave and complex event. Many of the responses have ignored the fact that in some settings, development simply cannot take place without consideration of this epidemic. All the gains, whether they are in education or agricultural production, are threatened by the southern African epidemic. It is quite unbelievable that the (realistic) assessment of the chances of reaching the MDGs should have such a blind spot when it comes to this disease.

There are no easy answers, either to HIV/AIDS itself, or to an understanding and response. What is desperately needed is a better understanding of what it means for development. This deconstruction of the nexus of development and HIV/AIDS will raise a question that can be answered best from a multidisciplinary perspective: what is the causal relationship between development and HIV? Only then, through a range of disciplines, can we begin to understand and then respond to the long-term impact of HIV/AIDS on development.

References

Africa Commission. 2005. *Our Common Interest: Report of the Commission for Africa*. Available at http://www.commissionforafrica.org, accessed 25 June 2006.

Barnett, Tony. 2006. 'A Long-Wave Event: HIV/AIDS, Politics, Governance and "Security": Sundering the Intergenerational Bond.' *International Affairs* 82(2): 297–313.

Barnett, Tony and Gwyn Prins. 2006. *HIV/AIDS and Security: Fact, Fiction and Evidence*. Geneva: UNAIDS; London: London School of Economics.

Barnett, Tony and Alan Whiteside. 2006. *AIDS in the Twenty-First Century: Disease and Globalization*. Hampshire and New York: Palgrave MacMillan.

Behrman, Greg. 2004. *The Invisible People*. New York: Free Press.

Black, Richard. 2005. 'Poverty and the World Summit'. *BBC News Analysis* 12 September. Available at http://news.bbc.co.uk, accessed 13 September 2005.

Bloom, David E. and Joyce V. Lyons (eds.). 1993. *Economic Implications of AIDS in Asia*. New Delhi: UNDP.

Campbell, Catherine. 2003. *Letting Them Die: Why HIV/AIDS Intervention Programmes Fail*. Oxford: James Currey.

Chazan, May. 2006. 'Seven Deadly Assumptions: Unravelling the Implications of HIV/AIDS among Grandmothers in Warwick Junction'. In *South Africa and Beyond*, draft manuscript.

Cohen, Des. 1992. *The Economic Impact of the HIV Epidemic*. Report of the United Nations Development Programme. New York: UNDP.

Cross, Sholto and Alan Whiteside (eds.). 1993. *Facing up to AIDS: The Socio-Economic Impact in Southern Africa*. London: Macmillan.

De Waal, Alex. 2006. *AIDS and Power: Why There Is No Political Crisis – Yet*. London and New York: Zed Books.

Fourie, Pieter. 2006. *The Political Management of HIV and AIDS in South Africa*. Basingstoke: Palgrave.

Gaolathe, Baledzi (Minister of Finance and Development Planning). 2002. 'Speech on Draft National Development Plan 9 (2003/2004–2008/2009) delivered to the Botswana National Assembly, 21 November'. Available at http://www.sarpn.org.za/documents/d0000257/P248_Development _Plan9.pdf, accessed 30 January 2008.

Gumede, William Mervin. 2005. *Thabo Mbeki and the Battle for the Soul of the ANC*. Cape Town: Zebra Press.

Halperin, Daniel T. and Helen Epstein. 2004. 'Concurrent Sexual Partnerships Help to Explain Africa's High HIV Prevalence: Implications for Prevention'. *The Lancet* 364 (9 428): 4–6.

Iliffe, John. 2006. *The African AIDS Epidemic: A History*. Oxford: James Currey.

Mann, Charles C. 2005. *Ancient Americans: Rewriting the History of the New World*. London: Granta Books.

Newell, Marie-Louise, Heena Brahmbhatt and Peter H. Ghys. 2004. 'Child Mortality and HIV Infection in Africa'. *AIDS* 18 (Supplement 2): S27–S34.

Office of the Presidency of South Africa. 2007. *Development Indicators, Mid-Term Review*, June. Tshwane: Office of the Presidency of South Africa.

Sewankambo, Nelson K., Ronald H. Gray, Saifuddin Ahmad, David Serwadda, Fred Wabwire-Mangen, Fred Nalugoda, Noah Kiwanuka, Tom Lutalo, and Godfrey Kigozi. 2000. 'Mortality Associated with HIV Infection in Rural Rakai District, Uganda'. *AIDS* 14(15): 391–400.

Shilts, Randy. 1988. *And the Band Played on: People, Politics and the AIDS Epidemic*. London: Viking.

Shisana, Olive, Tom Rehle, Leickness C. Simbayi, Warren Parker, Khangelani Zuma, A. Bhana, Cathy Connolly, Sean Jooste, Victoria Pillay, et al. 2005. *South African National HIV Prevalence, HIV Incidence, Behaviour and Communication Survey 2005*. Cape Town: Human Sciences Research Council Press.

Reproductive Health Research Unit. 2004. 'HIV and Sexual Behaviour among Young South Africans: A National Survey of 15–24-Year-Olds'. Johannesburg.

Stats SA (Statistics South Africa). 2006. *Mortality and Causes of Death in South Africa, 2003 and 2004: Findings from Death Notifications*. Statistical release, P0309.3, Pretoria.

UN (United Nations). 2000. 'Millennium Development Goals (MDGs)'. Available at http:// www.un.org/millenniumgoals/goals.html, accessed 7 July 2006.

———. 2005. *In Larger Freedom: Towards Development Security and Human Rights for All*. Report of the UN Secretary-General, A/59/2005, March.

———. 2007. *The Millennium Development Goals Report*. Available at http://www.un.org/ millenniumgoals/pdf/mdg2007.pdf, accessed 30 January 2008.

UNAIDS (Joint United Nations Programme on HIV/AIDS) and World Health Organisation (WHO). 2007. 'AIDS Epidemic Update'. December. UNAIDS/07.27E/JC1322E.

UN General Assembly. 2000. *United Nations Millennium Declaration*. Resolution adopted by the General Assembly, A/RES/55/2, September.

———. 2005a. 'Follow-up to the Outcome of the Millennium Summit'. Draft resolution to adopt the 2005 World Summit Outcome, 15 September. Available at http://www.un.org/summit 2005, accessed 25 June, 2006.

————. 2005b. '2005 World Summit Outcome'. A/RES/60/1. Available at http://www.daccessdds. un.org/doc/UNDOC/GEN/N05/510/94/PDF/N0551094.pdf?OpenElement, accessed 30 January 2008.

UN News Service. 2005. Various press releases, 16–20 September. Available at http://www.un.org/ summit, accessed 25 June 2006.

UNSC (United Nations Security Council). 2000. 'UNSC Resolution 1308, on the Responsibility of the Security Council in the Maintenance of International Peace and Security: HIV/AIDS and International Peace-Keeping Operations'. Adopted by the Security Council at its 4 172nd meeting, 17 July 2000.

UN Secretariat, Population Division, Department of Economic and Social Affairs. 2003. 'The Impact of AIDS'. 2 September. ESA/P/WP.

UN Statistics Division. 2005. *Progress towards the Millennium Development Goals, 1990–2005*. Available at http://www.unstats.un.org/unsd/mdg/Host.aspx?Content=Products/Progress 2005.htm, accessed 9 March 2008.

Whiteside, Alan. 2008. *HIV/AIDS: A Very Short Introduction*. Oxford: Oxford University Press.

World Bank. 1997. *Confronting AIDS: Public Priorities in a Global Epidemic*. Oxford: Oxford University Press.

11

The United Nations and the Securitisation of HIV/AIDS

———— • ————

Pieter Fourie

AIDS is a new type of global emergency – an unprecedented threat to human development requiring sustained action and commitment over the long term. (UN 2004, 7)

A quarter century of HIV and AIDS

On 5 June 1981, the Centre for Disease Control and Prevention (CDC) in the United States published its *Weekly Morbidity and Mortality Report*, chronicling for the first time the symptoms among a few urban gay men of what was set to become the most deadly disease known to humanity. That was over 25 years ago and since then, the HIV/AIDS pandemic has killed almost 30 million individuals worldwide.

According to the global report published by the Joint United Nations Programme on HIV/AIDS (UNAIDS) in mid-2006, some data for the proximate southern African region can be summarised as shown in Table 11.1.

This translates into more than 3 000 deaths among citizens of Southern African Development Community (SADC) states *every single day* – and this number is steadily increasing. To put this in comparative perspective, these numbers mean that SADC experiences the equivalent number of deaths of a 9/11 attack every single day of each year.

To make matters worse, epidemiologists tell us that the AIDS epidemic (since it results from HIV, a lentivirus, or slow-acting virus) is a 'long-wave event'. Among other implications, this means that we are faced with an insidious phenomenon that might take up to 50 or even 120 years to play itself out (Barnett 2006, 304; see

Table 11.1 HIV/AIDS prevalence in southern Africa (December 2005).

Country	Adults and children living with HIV	HIV prevalence (%) in adults aged 15–49	AIDS deaths (adults and children) in 2005	Number of orphans (0–17 years) due to AIDS
Angola	320 000	3.7	30 000	160 000
Botswana	270 000	24.1	18 000	120 000
DRC	1 000 000	3.2	90 000	680 000
Lesotho	270 000	23.2	23 000	97 000
Madagascar	49 000	0.5	2 900	13 000
Malawi	940 000	14.1	78 000	550 000
Mozambique	1 800 000	16.1	140 000	510 000
Namibia	230 000	19.6	17 000	85 000
South Africa	5 500 000	18.8	320 000	1 200 000
Swaziland	220 000	33.4	16 000	63 000
Tanzania	1 400 000	6.5	140 000	1 100 000
Zambia	1 100 000	17.0	98 000	710 000
Zimbabwe	1 700 000	20.1	180 000	1 100 000

Source: UNAIDS 2006, 500–40

also Chapter 10 in this volume). Nothing in human history is comparable with this and we simply do not know what the long-term impact of the pandemic will be.

How does one respond to such a threat in an effective and appropriately scaled way? A key response has been to polemicise the epidemic; a master narrative has been created to 'securitise' HIV/AIDS. By making appeals to states' security and by reconceptualising AIDS as an 'enemy' that needs to be 'battled' and 'defeated' (note the securocratic register or the language of war applied here), a number of effects can be achieved. These include the inculcation of a sense of imminent danger or threat, the creation of an identifiable and common villain, the rapid mobilisation of the required state/governmental resources required to respond to that threat, as well as myth-making about who the saviours or victors might be.

Since AIDS first made newspaper headlines in the early 1980s, this narrative or culture of securitisation has come to be associated with the epidemic and it is the purpose of this chapter to analyse the implications of such securitisation. In the context of the 'war against terror' after 11 September 2001, we are becoming increasingly familiar with the super-patriotic proclivities and nationalistic pathologies that securitisation can enable, so a closer look at the powerful constructivist role of specific conceptualisations of the pandemic is timely. One analyst observes that:

> In the aftermath of September 11, 2001, the United States tends to define all national security concerns through the prism of terrorism. That framework is overly limited even for the United States, and an absurdly narrow template to apply to the security of most other countries. The HIV/AIDS pandemic is aggravating a laundry list of underlying tensions in developing, declining, and failed states. As the burden of death due to HIV/AIDS skyrockets around the world over the next five to ten years, the disease may well play a more profound role on the security stage of many nations, and present the wealthy world with a challenge the likes of which it has never experienced. How countries, rich and poor, frame HIV/AIDS within their national security debates today may well determine how well they respond to the massive grief, demographic destruction, and security threats that the pandemic will present tomorrow. (Garrett 2005, 64)

There has, of course, been significant academic interest in the construction of metaphors and myths (including the notion of securitisation) of disease, including the HIV/AIDS epidemic in recent years (for example, see Elbe 2006; Altman 2003; Sontag 2002; Altman 1999; Fourie and Schönteich 2001; Heinecken 2001). This chapter attempts to highlight a rather interesting phenomenon of the last year or two: the growing introspection evident within UNAIDS. The United Nations (UN) is in crisis and searching desperately for, first, a *raison d'être* and greater relevance in the struggle against global threats in general and second, UNAIDS seems to be going through an important shift in its conceptualisation of this particular pandemic – and with regard to security. This is happening within the context of a mostly discreet, yet exceedingly influential battle between sovereign states set on preserving the right to determine their own responses to the epidemic and those pushing for the multilateralisation of responses to the pandemic. These multilateral responses include the World Bank's Millennium AIDS Programme (MAP), the US President's Emergency Programme for AIDS Relief (PEPFAR), as well as the Global Fund to Fight HIV/AIDS, Tuberculosis and Malaria (GFATM) initiatives (not to mention UNAIDS itself).

The scene is set for great tension between autonomous, state-centred interventions, on the one hand and these multilateral initiatives, on the other hand. Discursively, one of the ways in which this tension has manifested has been through appeals to either a (hard) securitisation agenda centred on the dangers that HIV/

AIDS implies for state survival, or an agenda that appeals more directly to a softer, human security approach, which underscores the threat to individual human rights posed by the epidemic. The latter approach has been most closely associated with a developmental agenda.

Avoiding an orthodox conceptual analysis, this chapter demonstrates how the concept of 'security' has evolved by focusing on the evolution of the UN within the context of this modern plague. The chapter's findings are counter-intuitive: as becomes clear in the course of the next few pages, the desperate introspection within this multilateral body post-11/9 (9 November 1989: the fall of the Berlin Wall) and post-9/11 (the terrorist attacks on the United States in September 2001) has led UNAIDS to adopt a potentially exciting ideological marriage between a traditional, militaristic way of thinking about security and the more contemporary, human security perspective alluded to above. The result of this confluence is the partial assertion of a new research agenda in terms of the UN and security, which will be discussed towards the end of the chapter.

Until now, most theorists have gone for an either/or approach: contrasting orthodox (militarist) and human security conceptions as mutually exclusive and then applying these to the pandemic. However, this chapter demonstrates that AIDS might very well be the catalyst for a significant institutional change within the UN. The exclusivist conceptual approach might be falling away, leading not to greater relativism or facile, postmodern permissiveness, but to a useful marriage of ideas about security that could inform the UN's perception of its role in the world, as well as the way in which national and international actors respond to long-wave events, such as the HIV/AIDS epidemic. Finally, this chapter illustrates this change by evaluating the findings of a recent scenario-building project, titled *AIDS in Africa: Three Scenarios to 2025* (UNAIDS and WHO 2005).

Changing global conceptions of security

In power politics – politically, as well as economically – words and institutions matter and these have had significant impacts on the manner in which ideologies have shaped elites' mental maps, descriptions and prescriptions about the allocation of scarce resources in broader society. The multilateralisation of AIDS as a security issue has recently come into its own: 'the intervention of the Security Council in 2000 was a critical move in securitising HIV/AIDS, *constructing* the disease as something extraordinary which demanded international attention and action'

(McInnes 2006, 315; emphasis added). In these terms, the current global order is the result of three major ideological developments that inform everything from international law to the way in which multilateral institutions and states conceptualise and respond to new threats such as HIV/AIDS.

The first major ideological development was the Treaty of Westphalia of 1648, which ended the 30-year religious war in Europe and established the modern state system. Modern notions of state sovereignty and the search for a global balance of power in the absence of a global government resulted from this development and continue to permeate the way in which states relate to each other. Normatively, the realist ideology that emanated from the Treaty of Westphalia emphasises the centrality of state's autonomy and security – notions that have become embedded in international law and inform how governments, in particular, respond to external and other threats.

This realist notion of traditional security has since been questioned, and in some ways challenged, by liberal notions of global power (see Chapter 1 in this volume). The French Revolution of 1789 shifted the state-centric view towards greater empathy for a humanistic and individually based level of analysis. The state was now seen as complementary to the interests of its citizens, whose rights it was obligated to protect. These notions have also become embedded in international law and other institutions – including UN conventions on individual human rights (among which are rights to health and other forms of security). This human-centred approach was further supported by the more developmental focus emphasised by Marxist thinkers, who conceptualise security and what it is that we need to be safe from, according to the original writings of Karl Marx and others in the mid-to-late nineteenth century. Rather than focusing on the individual unit of analysis, as liberals would, proponents of Marxism underline the importance of economic class and exploitation resulting from material inequalities and structural deficiencies at both national and global levels.

This bit of ideological history is important, as it has had a direct impact on the evolution of the UN as a potential custodian of peace and security after the Second World War. The victors at the end of the War wanted to create an organisation that would assist in establishing a global order based on the notion of 'collective security'. States would become each other's keepers to prevent any individual member of the UN from exploiting economic or politically nationalistic notions and dragging the world into a third world war (Nye 2000). This new system of collective security was entrenched institutionally through the creation of the UN, whose policies were couched in terms of an evolving global legal system based broadly on guarantees of state sovereignty, collective state security and individual human rights. The ideal thus became a rather interesting hybrid of realist and liberal discourses applied within the multilateral organisation, with members of especially the new Second and Third Worlds emphasising (discursively at least) notions of greater global class equity and fairness. The post-Second-World-War, multilateral context thus created a political arena in which the three main ideologies (realism, liberalism and Marxism) pertaining to evolving notions of 'security' could be tested and played out.

The difficulties that this implied within the cold-war context are interesting, but fall outside of the ambit of this chapter. After 1989 and the end of that ideological conflict, however, the UN needed to seriously reconsider its conception of security. No longer was the world subject to the conventional notions of conflict and other threats that permeated the orthodox description of realpolitik. The global context had moved on from the narrow ideological battle between the First and Second Worlds, which had mostly played out in Third World proxy wars. After 1989, nationalism reasserted itself: from intrastate conflicts in the Balkans and in Africa to the appearance of a new kind of terrorism wrought of fundamentalist or politicised religions. Interestingly, it was also around the same time (in 1990) that the US Central Intelligence Agency (CIA) first identified HIV/AIDS as a variable that might cause greater state fragility and eventual failure, particularly in the developing world (Fourie and Schönteich 2002, 8). As traditional, military notions of security threats started to recede in the early 1990s, the UN Development Programme (UNDP) released its Human Development Report, in which it coined the term 'human security', taken to refer to any threat (military or other) that undermines the well-being of humans (UNDP 1994).

The UN moved swiftly to put this new conception of security on the development agenda. Academia and other intellectuals responded predictably, by commencing an abstract and, in retrospect, rather predictably semantic game of establishing the different implications of a human security versus a military security agenda. These debates crystallised around two main positions. Most argued that the securitisation of an issue was useful, as it forced states to put issues such as HIV/AIDS on the public agenda. By applying the language of wars or imminent threat, states are able to mobilise resources. As Colin McInnes argues, 'there is more than a suspicion that the securitising move [within the UN] was part of an attempt to gain greater political attention for the HIV/AIDS crisis' (2006, 326). Other analysts warned that securitisation might actually have a counter-productive effect: by 'othering' and 'enemising' selective aspects of the pandemic (for example: homosexuals, sex workers, injecting drug users, insidious 'big pharma.' and so on), the securitisation of the epidemic could serve to increase stigmatisation of people living with HIV/AIDS (PLWHA) (see Elbe 2006; Sontag 2002).

Be that as it may, in the short term, the securitisation of AIDS achieved exactly what many said it needed to. In December 1999, the US ambassador to the UN, Richard Holbrooke, visited Africa to personally witness the impact of the growing HIV/AIDS epidemic. On 10 January 2000, the UN Security Council debated what was ostensibly a health issue in security terms, for the first time in its history (Behrman 2004, 158–65). This meeting was followed in July 2000 by the adoption of UN Resolution 1 308, which formalised the securitisation of HIV/AIDS (UNSC 2000). It is important that these developments took place within the Security Council: in the days of the cold war, this was the UN body where global powers could do their posturing – the Security Council is a state-centric vehicle par excellence. However, Resolution 1 308 invoked much of the language of human security, as it formally securitised the pandemic and UNAIDS was charged with responding to the challenge.

This was a significant victory for UNAIDS, which was established (as successor to the Global Programme on AIDS) 'in 1996 after a bloody four-year battle for control within the UN "family"' (Hunter 2003, 38). UNAIDS is not an autonomous UN agency, but rather a secretariat attempting to build consensus on a particular issue (HIV/AIDS) among a range of other (territorially jealous) UN agencies – not an easy task by any stretch of the imagination. Dennis Altman observes that UNAIDS is caught in a contradiction it cannot resolve: its success depends on establishing co-operation between the UN agencies that are its co-sponsors, where territorial claims are often more important than policy outcomes. For UNAIDS to co-ordinate, say, the World Bank and the UN Educational, Scientific and Cultural Organisation (UNESCO) is rather akin to asking a sparrow to direct a herd of elephants (Altman 2003).

However, Resolution 1 308 gave UNAIDS more of the institutional legitimacy it needed to act. One year after Resolution 1 308, in mid-2001, the UN General Assembly held a special session on HIV/AIDS (UNGASS), which went even further in putting the pandemic on the multilateral agenda. During the special session, former US Military Chief of Staff and then Secretary of State, General Colin Powell, declared that 'there is no enemy in war more insidious than AIDS' (cited in Behrman

2004, 266). The UNAIDS secretariat has had some amazing successes. For instance, considering specifically military aspects of UN operations, Laurie Garrett notes that:

> All military personnel stationed with UN operations are by regulation encouraged to undergo voluntary HIV screening. In addition, the UN's roughly 47 000 peacekeepers all receive training about the risks of AIDS, other sexually transmitted diseases, and appropriate behaviour with civilian personnel. They also all get a plastic 'HIV/AIDS Awareness Card for Peacekeeping Operations' and five or six condoms a week during foreign deployment. Most of the 65 000 peacekeepers perform their work with noble courage and free of HIV risk. (2005, 56)

UN introspection regarding AIDS and security

UNAIDS has also done some intellectual soul-searching. Anyone who has worked within the UN system can attest to the fact that the minutiae of bureaucratic politics can at times be frustrating. However, UNAIDS has moved fairly swiftly and effectively and in 2003, worked with Royal Dutch/Shell in London to build a set of future scenarios on the impact of the HIV/AIDS pandemic on Africa over the next twenty years. UNAIDS has also liaised with external partners in the AIDS, Security and Conflict Initiative (ASCI), which has been assisting the UN in its identification of a new research and policy agenda, particularly with regard to more traditional security issues. The results of ASCI are to be made public by 2008.

UNAIDS has also participated in three further seminal reports. The first is the report of the Secretary-General's High-Level Panel on Threats, Challenges and Change (UN 2004). Significantly, Kofi Annan, then the UN Secretary-General, used the foreword to the High-Level Panel report to reiterate the central role of states in combating today's security threats, thus emphasising the realist underpinnings of the modern global state system and the concomitant implications for the definition and locus of security that this invokes: 'the front line in today's combat must be manned by capable and responsible *States*' (UN 2004, vii). However, in the next two paragraphs, Annan qualifies such realism by reflecting on the human security obligations that such a role implies for sovereign states – in relation to what he calls 'development' and 'biological security'.

The High-Level Panel report is thus quite explicit in its suggestion of a new security consensus – one which does not state the conceptualisation of 'security' in either hard versus soft, or state versus human security terms:

> The central challenge for the twenty-first century is to fashion a new
> and broader understanding, bringing together all these strands, of what
> collective security means – and of all the responsibilities, commitments,
> strategies and institutions that come with it if a collective security system
> is to be effective, efficient and equitable . . . What is needed today is
> nothing less than a new consensus between alliances that are frayed,
> between wealthy nations and poor, and among peoples mired in mistrust
> across an apparently widening cultural abyss. The essence of that
> consensus is simple: we all share responsibility for each other's security.
> And the test of that consensus will be action . . . Any event or process
> that leads to large-scale death or lessening of life chances and
> undermines States as the basic unit of the international system is a
> threat to international security. (UN 2004, 1–2)

The UN appears to be working towards making peace with the ostensible tension
between state sovereignty and post-Second-World-War multilateralism by unequivocally accepting the state as the global unit of analysis (Gray 2005, 212), while
at the same time drawing special attention to the obligations that states have to
protect individuals' rights to health and safety. Not since the original
conceptualisation of the traditional collective security agenda in the first half of the
twentieth century has the UN gone through such an explicit process of introspection
about a concept that it uses to motivate for programmatic action against threats
such as the global HIV/AIDS epidemic.

The second important report that UNAIDS commissioned in order to refine its
own conception of, and response to, security issues was published in March 2006.
Entitled *HIV/AIDS and Security: Fact, Fiction and Evidence*, the report is the first serious
effort to find empirical data that links the pandemic to global security issues –
particularly security issues related to uniformed personnel (peacekeepers are included
in this category, but it generally refers to the military and police). The authors of
the report found that many of the purported causal and other links between
insecurity and HIV/AIDS are simply unsubstantiated. Since the late 1990s, there
has been a growing intellectual industry producing conjecture on this subject, but
the evidence consists of what the authors call 'factoids': one researcher simply quotes
another and soon opinions morph into dogma. This manner of securitising AIDS
has had the consequence that 'regardless of motivation, the resultant rising political

priority has worked to foreclose prematurely the research phase in a rush to define responses' (Barnett and Prins 2006, 360).

The latter is one of the dangers of securitisation, namely unwanted consequences in terms of the construction of an environment that highlights, dramatises and embraces hasty response exigencies: '. . . that perverse potential to induce consequences opposite to those intended subvert the required cycle of validation of outcome upon which confidence in the correctness of a decision largely depends' (Barnett and Prins 2006, 361). In other words, the need to research, constantly analyse and refine responses may at times get lost in the rush to act on alarming, but not necessarily well-founded, early conclusions about the scale and nature of the threats posed by HIV.

The report found that despite the statements to the contrary, there is virtually no empirical evidence on the relationship between HIV/AIDS and uniformed services. We know very little about how HIV/AIDS impacts on the operational readiness of standing armies, what the implications are for international burden-sharing in peacemaking and peacekeeping operations, or the human resources issues that accompany these variables (see Chapter 9 in this volume). The report highlights an urgent need for better empirical research on the supposed implications of HIV/AIDS for the uniformed services. It argues that a new agenda regarding security should incorporate a new research agenda for issues peripheral to the ostensibly more semantic core of this complex issue.

In late 2005, an important internal report was compiled for UNAIDS by Laetitia van den Assum, a senior Dutch diplomat on secondment to the office of Dr Peter Piot (executive director of UNAIDS). The report deals explicitly with how UNAIDS and the greater UN family should conceptualise and deal with the security implications of the HIV/AIDS pandemic. The document is of critical importance as it stems from UNAIDS's internal recognition that it needs to rethink its entire take on the AIDS-security nexus. It was also written at the same time as the *Fact, Fiction and Evidence* document discussed above and within the context of a short succession of formal intra-UN resolutions and debates about security at a macro-level. Some of the key findings of the Van den Assum document, entitled 'Towards a UNAIDS Framework Agenda for AIDS and Security', are as follows:

- Capturing the interplay between AIDS and security requires a broader and more inclusive concept of security, one that is human-centric (i.e. liberal), but at the same time recognises states' obligations to guarantee citizens' security (i.e. realism) (Van den Assum 2005, 2). The implication is that the UN, or at least UNAIDS, should avoid reducing the required response to AIDS and insecurity to a decision between either state-centric or developmentalist/ human security approaches. The statement is also significant in that it emphasises the obligations that accompany sovereignty within a state-centric global order – in this case, an obligation to protect citizens against the threat and impacts of AIDS (2005, 6-7).

• Given the combination of short-term shocks and long-term challenges associated with the epidemic, a combination of 'development relief' and 'emergency development' is needed to address the new type of emergency caused by HIV/AIDS (2005, 2-3). This incorporates the reality that HIV/AIDS is a long-wave event and recognises that we simply do not yet know how the pandemic will impact in the decades ahead. It creates room for a long-term emergency response, rather than short-term and possibly counter-productive interventions.

Conceptually as well as programmatically, this intellectual development can have significant implications for the way in which the UN responds to AIDS and other threats to security, since, as noted above, a 'threat to security' is now defined as 'any event or process that leads to large-scale death or lessening of life chances and undermines States as the basic unit of the international system' (UN 2004). The report emphasises the importance of the outcome of the ongoing ASCI project, which promises to combine empirical evidence on how these variables interact with appropriate policy guidelines.

Most recently – in late May and early June 2006 – the UN hosted UNGASS II, a summit held to mark the 25th anniversary of the first documented HIV/AIDS cases. This meeting was attended by 151 nations in New York and sought to update the UNGASS 2001 declaration that provided the momentum for a worldwide campaign against AIDS. Going into the summit, UNAIDS hoped to get states to agree on commitments and numerical targets to increase spending from the current US$8.2 billion per year for fighting AIDS to US$22 billion annually by 2010 (Piot 2006). However, the US administration blocked these and other key proposals because of its opposition to needle exchanges and references in the proposals to sex workers, injecting drug users and homosexuals. The United States found support from a number of African countries (including South Africa, Egypt and Gabon), who rejected numerical targets and thus the African Common Position, approved one month earlier by African Union (AU) heads of state in preparation for UNGASS II. The summit ended with agreement on a much watered-down text (UNGASS 2006), with vague references to numerical commitments (and hence no way of holding governments accountable) and 'coy references to high-risk groups' (*Guardian Unlimited* 2006).

UNAIDS, scenarios and future security in Africa

As noted previously, the AIDS pandemic is a long-wave event, which might last anything between 50 and 120 years. The conventional parameters of such an event and the best possible programmatic responses to such a crisis in slow motion are simply unknown, as has been indicated in the foregoing section regarding thinking about the AIDS-security nexus. Such long-wave events share a number of distinguishing features:

- one is usually unaware of their starting point;
- once awareness is there, it is difficult to reverse the progress and impact of the long-wave crisis/event;
- people with power (such as politicians) find it difficult to face such crises, since their own terms in office or power are much shorter and it is difficult to consistently mobilise resources appropriate to the crisis over the long term;
- there are few precedents for such events, which means that there is little experience or best practice to fall back on – leading to a sense of fatalism and impotence;
- such events tend to overwhelm even the most whole-hearted of government strategies;
- hastily conceived short-term responses may turn out to have been band-aid solutions that actually undermine more effective, longer-term responses, and
- a holistic response to such long-wave events requires long-term thinking that challenges the contemporary short-term way of doing things among current epistemic and political elites. (Barnett 2006, 302–03)

So how can we get beyond this last hurdle, in particular, and start to combine a solution-oriented way of looking at AIDS with a long view? How will AIDS impact on Africa's security? How can we become more secure on this most affected continent? How does UNAIDS see its own conceptions of security evolving over the next few decades? What factors will drive Africa and the world's responses to the AIDS epidemic, and what kind of future will there be for the next generation? It is precisely this last question that a recent UNAIDS research project attempts to answer. The report entitled *AIDS in Africa: Three Scenarios to 2025* was published in 2005 and despite some significant problems (see Fourie 2004, 54–59; Barnett 2006, 311–13), the scenarios project yielded some fascinating insights.

Scenarios methodologies are used to evoke innovative thinking about the future. This is not the future based on a single set of assumptions about the present (for that would be mere forecasting, or at most, educated guessing about what lies ahead), but rather a set of futures based on different assumptions about the present, presented with the different paths that might be taking us to these alternative futures (for more about scenario methodologies and futures studies, see Kahane 2004; Schwartz 1996, 2003; Van der Heijden 1996; De Geus 1998; Wack 1985a, 1985b). Such qualitative analysis is combined with quantitative methodologies and the different sets of assumptions are modelled by economists, demographers, actuaries, and so on. The key strength of future scenarios is that they show what *might* happen, rather than what we *want* to happen – they help us to move beyond our own mental maps, to think the unthinkable and to plan accordingly. In short, scenario-building implies choice – and therefore hope. The UNAIDS/WHO project developed three scenarios of how HIV and AIDS might impact on Africa between 2005 and 2025 (2005).

Scenario one: Tough choices

The first scenario presents a story in which African leaders choose to take tough measures that reduce the spread of HIV in the long term, even if it means difficulties in the short term. Leaders and communities work together, rather than against each other, in order to legitimise policy measures that might be unpopular. This is an Africa in which the state or government is seen to be more important than (especially Western) notions of individual human rights: the state intervenes unilaterally, rather than kowtowing to outside insistence on so-called 'best practice' – for instance, women are 'protected', rather than given greater freedom.

As resources are finite, governments target prevention, rather than ostensibly more expensive treatment strategies, making appeals to cultural traditions, rather than implementing a human rights-centred approach for the sake of global popularity or Eurocentric political correctness. Given the outside world's perpetual failure to ensure that donations actually reach the poorest of the poor, the West's 'donor and AIDS fatigue' vis-à-vis Africa as a whole and its shifting attention to Eastern Europe and Asia, the focus locally turns towards nation-building and more patriotic tendencies, rather than impotent attempts to please the global powers that be via increasing globalisation (which does not benefit Africa in any case) (UNAIDS and WHO 2005).

This is clearly an Africa where the militarist conception of security holds sway over a more developmental or human security-centred focus. The discourse of human security might be applied, particularly by African elites, but this is a secondary concern, one that is embedded within traditional notions of 'security'. Given finite resources, peacekeepers and other uniformed services receive preferential treatment in the allocation of resources to combat HIV/AIDS. Dissent is dealt with swiftly and mostly without regard for notions protective of individual human rights.

Scenario two: Traps and legacies

The second scenario tells a story in which Africa as a whole fails to escape from its more negative legacies. AIDS deepens the traps of poverty, underdevelopment and marginalisation in a globalising world. This is an Africa in which deep colonial divisions remain, at times leading to violent conflict at the interstate and intrastate level.

The cycle of poverty and AIDS becomes endemic across the region and as one country after another succumbs to the pressures wrought by the epidemic, governance structures collapse, sending the region as a whole into a collective whirlpool of anarchy. Governments find it increasingly difficult to invest in longer-term interventions against the HIV/AIDS epidemic, eventually leading to short-term and quick-fix solutions that benefit no one. Self-serving HIV/AIDS industries siphon off the few resources that are available for battling the epidemic: for instance, organised crime networks steal and smuggle antiretroviral (ARV) medicines across the continent, undermining their effective and appropriate dissemination. Africa becomes increasingly marginalised from the rest of the globalising world – except for those parts of especially oil-rich states that are bought up and controlled by foreigners, with energy profits leaving the African continent for foreign shores. Private armies guard any commodities that foreign multinational corporations hold in Africa.

As in other countries in southern Africa, in South Africa, vast sections outside the main urban centres would become ungovernable in the absence of a coherent central administrative order. Towards the end of the scenario timeline, Africa is supremely aid-dependent, but overseas development assistance is in increasingly short supply; the outside world has given up on Africa (UNAIDS and WHO 2005).

This is a future where human rights-centred approaches are viewed with cynicism or outright rejection. It is a dog-eat-dog world where only the strongest and the fittest might survive and traditional, militaristic conceptions of the link between AIDS and security remain the orthodoxy and notions of human security seem anachronistic and out of place – a luxury.

Scenario three: Times of transition

The third and final scenario tells the story of what might happen if all of today's good intentions were translated into the coherent and integrated development response necessary to tackle HIV and AIDS in Africa. The HIV/AIDS epidemic creates a global perception of crisis – one that is concerned not only about disease and global health apartheid, but all issues of global inequity. AIDS thus becomes a catalyst for a truly global transformation.

The result is the rapid and worldwide roll-out of treatment and prevention strategies: large pharmaceutical companies relinquish their intellectual property rights on ARVs and other life-saving drugs and an active civil society works with governments to roll out comprehensive AIDS regimens. National policy responses focus on reducing poverty, which is one of the main vectors of all epidemics. Africa and external partners democratise institutions such as the World Trade Organisation (WTO), the International Monetary Fund (IMF), the World Bank and the UN in order to fast-track key changes in global trade, especially, and in conflict prevention to promote peace and security. As time goes by, critical changes in male-female relations mean that men stop hiding behind notions of 'culture' in order to rationalise and perpetuate inequality and death (UNAIDS and WHO 2005).

This is a future in which the current new research agenda and contemporary reconceptualisation of the HIV/AIDS-security link have not only become the new orthodoxy, but have also galvanised sufficient support to catalyse changes across Africa and globally. The new security agenda is that traditional and human rights approaches to HIV/AIDS and security are no longer antithetical and constitute a paradoxical gift of the pandemic. HIV/AIDS provides Africans, as well as global elites, with a wholly novel way of viewing crises, enabling social learning about what it means to be secure, what it means to be a caring global society and how to achieve a more just and fairer global environment. The UN becomes one of the key implementers, as well as institutional and moral custodian of this new global order.

Scenarios enable most insight when they are read as a unit and comparatively: the main qualitative modalities of the three UNAIDS scenarios can be summarised as in Table 11.2.

Table 11.2   HIV/AIDS scenarios in Africa (2005–25).

Branching points	Tough choices	Traps and legacies	Times of transition
How is the crisis perceived?	AIDS is but one manifestation of a broad development crisis.	Largely as a medical crisis. HIV is tackled in isolation from its social and economic context.	AIDS is a metaphor for global crisis.
And by whom?	African leaders.	By many, but no effective, co-ordinated action.	Civil society, Africa and the global community.
Will there be the incentive to address the crisis?	Yes. Although HIV is seen as one of many challenges.	Yes. However, funding drives a so-called 'AIDS industry'.	Yes. AIDS is a key catalyst for a reconfiguration of international and national priorities.
And the capacity?	Yes. Major national efforts to rebuild capacity to respond to the epidemic. Key emphasis on prevention and antiretroviral therapy to maintain essential capacity.	No. High level of resources initially leads to wasteful duplication and uncoordinated efforts. AIDS strips the capacity to respond in high HIV prevalence countries.	Yes. Major mobilising of national and international resources.

Source: UNAIDS and WHO 2005, 58

The UN's new security agenda: Where to now?

There are two critical points that need to be considered by the research and policy communities in formulating their priorities for the future.

Words matter

How HIV/AIDS – the 'problem' – is defined, and by whom, will make a fundamental difference in terms of how responses to the pandemic are conceptualised and implemented at both national and global levels (Ostergard and Barcelo 2005). The HIV/AIDS policy environment in South Africa, for example, is in disarray because of contending and contested definition spaces (Fourie 2006; see also Chapters 2, 3 and 4 in this volume). As demonstrated above, the UN itself is coming to grips with the rapidly shifting ontological demands that the pandemic implies. On a continental level, Africa needs to find its own voice regarding perceptions and conceptualisations of the purported links between AIDS and security (De Waal 2003) – the UNAIDS/WHO future scenarios project has made it abundantly clear that outside multilateral agendas cannot effectively be projected into any context.

Reliable numbers matter

Inductive research can all too quickly lead intellectual elites into a trap of 'tail-wags-the-dog' or 'factoidal' result-seeking. Malleable conceptual clarity requires action based on reliable empirical evidence and the AIDS research community has seen precious little of this. The result is that we have been at war with each other over semantics and dollars, rather than united against the HIV/AIDS pandemic. Researchers everywhere – including in the institutions of the UN – need to be more accountable to the clients implied by contemporary conceptions of the marriage between heterodox conceptions of security.

Conclusion

With these two broad insights in mind, a number of specific research areas requiring urgent enquiry into the link between AIDS and security present themselves. These include the need for:

- Better data: more and better data should be collected on the impact and implications of the epidemic for government departments. An integrated surveillance system should be established for recording rates of HIV and AIDS in uniformed services, within obvious constraints of confidentiality and security. Data should be collected on the demographic structure of armies and other uniformed services, their experiences with ARV medicines, terms of access for serving members and their households, and service policies in relation to HIV/AIDS issues in general. The implications of HIV/AIDS for force strength should also be analysed (for more on this issue in South Africa, see Chapter 9 in this volume).

The impact and implications of the epidemic for governance, particularly governmental service provision and vital public functions, should also be explored. Such research should examine not only the consequences of the epidemic for the delivery of basic services, but also implications of HIV/AIDS in prison settings (see Chapter 8 in this volume) and its likely effects on judicial and court systems, with a view to establishing strategies to mitigate the effects of the epidemic for government institutions. There is further need for careful research to test the hypothesis that HIV/AIDS threatens state stability and may cause civil unrest and rising levels of crime and violence (see Chapter 7 in this volume). Scenario-building and other methodologies should be used to explore the possible impact of HIV/AIDS on security and to expand thinking about this and other long-wave events.

- New approaches to governance: stakeholders must recognise the new type of emergency presented by HIV/AIDS in high-prevalence countries and develop policies and programmes designed to counter this trend, as well as to mitigate the impact on communities, service providers and vital public sector functions. There is little consensus on what good governance entails in the context of the epidemic. This also points to the need to establish an agenda for HIV/AIDS and governance, including HIV/AIDS governance within public sector institutions.

- Research into HIV/AIDS in the uniformed services: in addition to the more general research on the implications of the HIV/AIDS epidemic for militaries and other uniformed services, there is a need for research into the availability of prevention, treatment and care and support programmes in military institutions and the police and how these can be improved to better mitigate the effects of the epidemic. Such data should be used to inform the integration of prevention, diagnostic, treatment and care services for households and families of military and other uniformed service personnel, while paying particular attention to gender issues (see Chapter 9 in this volume). The question of how HIV/AIDS is being addressed in the context of security sector reforms, rule of law and rape in relation to concentrations of uniformed service populations should also be examined.

While it is widely argued that HIV/AIDS will increasingly influence peacekeeping and the maintenance of more traditional notions of security, there is little information on the implications of HIV/AIDS for peacekeeping. This suggests the need for focused research into both the implications of the epidemic for troop-contributing countries' ability to deploy troops to peace-keeping missions and the risk of troops contracting and transmitting HIV while on a mission. The relationship between the uniformed services and their host environments should be explored, both at home and on missions. Detailed ethnographic studies of deployed personnel's behaviour, particularly risky sexual behaviour, should be conducted and the relationship between sexual risk-taking and military training explored. The implications of HIV/AIDS for international burden-sharing in peace enforcement, peacemaking and peacekeeping among UN member states should also be established.

• Better practice within the UN system: UNAIDS should continue to engage with regional organisations such as the AU, the Economic Community of West African States (ECOWAS) and SADC. There is also scope for greater engagement with and among UN co-sponsors on HIV/AIDS issues. UNAIDS should continue to advocate AIDS mainstreaming in multilateral policy and planning instruments, including, in particular, poverty reduction strategy papers (PRSPs). Ongoing UNAIDS programmes with uniformed services should be reviewed. UNAIDS should also collaborate with the UN Peace Building Support Office (PBSO) to ensure that AIDS-related needs receive high priority as an integral part of UN peace-building efforts. (Barnett and Prins 2006; Benatar 2005; Netherlands Ministry of Foreign Affairs 2005; Van den Assum 2005)

Overall, analysts in general and the UN, in particular, should be wary of notions invoking any so-called 'tyranny of best practice': HIV/AIDS is not a monolithic epidemic; it has a variety of impacts in different localities. Thus intervention must move away from a 'one-size-fits-all approach into much smarter and more targeted policies and programmes' (Netherlands Ministry of Foreign Affairs 2005, 2). That said, the global HIV/AIDS pandemic allows us an unprecedented opportunity for societal and intellectual learning and can go beyond being, as it is to many onlookers, an assemblage of tragic anecdotes to become a truly transformational social agent. But in order to get there, we as researchers and policy-makers need to address the issues outlined above. Perhaps HIV/AIDS is not the problem; rather, it is the symptom of other structural global problems that determine the patterns and events of everyday lives and the key lesson is that we need to fix our world. We are only 25 years into this long-wave event; these are early days yet, but the clock is ticking.

References

Altman, Dennis. 1999. 'AIDS and Questions of Global Governance'. *Pacifica Review* 11, 2 June: 195–211.

———. 2003. 'HIV and Security'. *International Relations* 17(4): 417–27.

Barnett, Tony. 2006. 'A Long-Wave Event: HIV/AIDS, Politics, Governance and "Security": Sundering the Intergenerational Bond?' *International Affairs* 82(2): 297–313.

Barnett, Tony and Gwyn Prins. 2006. *HIV/AIDS and Security: Fact, Fiction and Evidence*. Geneva: UNAIDS; London: London School of Economics. Also published in *International Affairs* 82(2): 359–68 (page references in this chapter refer to this publication).

Behrman, Greg. 2004. *The Invisible People: How the US Has Slept through the Global AIDS Pandemic, the Greatest Humanitarian Catastrophe of Our Time*. New York and London: Free Press.

Benatar, Solomon. 2005. 'The HIV/AIDS Pandemic: A Sign of Instability in a Complex Global System'. In *Ethics and AIDS in Africa: The Challenge to Our Thinking*, ed. Anton van Niekerk and Loretta Kopelman. Cape Town: David Philip.

De Geus, Arie. 1998. 'Planning as Learning'. *Harvard Business Review*, March–April: 70–74.

De Waal, Alex. 2003. 'Human Rights Organizations and the Political Imagination: How the West and Africa Have Diverged'. *Journal of Human Rights* 2(4), December: 475–94.

Elbe, Stefan. 2006. 'Should HIV/AIDS be Securitised? The Ethical Dilemmas of Linking HIV/AIDS and Security'. *International Studies Quarterly* 50(1): 119–44.

Fourie, Pieter. 2004. 'Multi-Stakeholders with Multiple Perspectives: HIV/AIDS in Africa'. *Development* 47(4): 54–59.

———. 2006. *The Political Management of HIV and AIDS in South Africa: One Burden Too Many?* Basingstoke and New York: Palgrave Macmillan.

Fourie, Pieter and Martin Schönteich. 2001. 'Africa's New Security Threat'. *African Security Review* 10(4): 29–57.

———. 2002. 'Die, the Beloved Countries: Human Security and HIV/AIDS in Africa'. *Politeia* 21(2): 6–30.

Garrett, Laurie. 2005. 'The Lessons of HIV/AIDS'. *Foreign Affairs* 84(4): 51–64.

Gray, Christine. 2005. 'Peacekeeping and Enforcement Action in Africa: The Role of Europe and the Obligations of Multilateralism'. *Review of International Studies* 31: 207–23.

Guardian Unlimited. 2006. 'US Blocking Deal on Fighting AIDS'. Published in *Mail & Guardian* 2 June. Available at http://www.mg.co.za/articlePage.aspx?articleid=273524&area=/breaking_news/breaking_news_international_news/, accessed 22 July 2006.

Heinecken, Lindy. 2001. 'Living in Terror: The Looming Security Threat to Southern Africa'. *African Security Review* 10(4): 7–17.

Hunter, Susan. 2003. *Who Cares? AIDS in Africa*. New York: Palgrave Macmillan.

Kahane, Adam. 2004. *Solving Tough Problems*. San Francisco: Berrett-Koehler.

McInnes, Colin. 2006. 'HIV/AIDS and Security'. *International Affairs* 82(2): 315–26.

Netherlands Ministry of Foreign Affairs. 2005. *AIDS, Security and Conflict Initiative*. Summary of briefing held on 3 June 2005 at the Dutch Mission, New York.

Nye, Joseph. 2000. *Understanding International Conflicts: An Introduction to Theory and History*. New York: Longman.

Ostergard, Robert and Crystal Barcelo. 2005. 'Personalist Regimes and the Insecurity Dilemma: Prioritising AIDS as a National Security Threat in Uganda'. In *The African State and the AIDS Crisis*, ed. Amy Patterson. Aldershot: Ashgate.

Piot, Peter. 2006. 'Statement at the UN General Assembly High Level Meeting on AIDS'. 31 May, New York.

Schwartz, Peter. 1996. *The Art of the Long View: Planning for the Future in an Uncertain World*. New York: Currency Doubleday.

———. 2003. *Inevitable Surprises: A Survival Guide for the 21st Century*. London: The Free Press.

Sontag, Susan. 2002. *Illness as Metaphor and AIDS and Its Metaphors*. London: Penguin Classics.

UN (United Nations). 2004. *A More Secure World: Our Shared Responsibility*. Report of the Secretary-General's High-Level Panel on Threats, Challenges and Change, UN, A/59/565, December.

———. 2006. 'General Assembly Resolution: Political Declaration on HIV/AIDS'. United Nations General Assembly Special Session II (UNGASS II) Declaration, Resolution 60/262, 2 June.

UNAIDS (Joint United Nations Programme on HIV/AIDS). 2006. 'Report on the Global AIDS Epidemic'. UNAIDS/06.20E.

UNAIDS (Joint United Nations Programme on HIV/AIDS) and WHO (World Health Organisation). 2005. *AIDS in Africa: Three Scenarios to 2025*. Geneva: UNAIDS and WHO.

UNDP (United Nations Development Programme). 1994. *New Dimensions of Human Security*. Human Development Report. Available at http://www.hdr.undp.org/reports/global/ 1994/en/, accessed 2 May 2007.

UNSC (United Nations Security Council). 2000. 'UNSC Resolution 1308, on the Responsibility of the Security Council in the Maintenance of International Peace and Security: HIV/AIDS and International Peace-Keeping Operations'. Adopted by the Security Council at its 4 172nd meeting, 17 July 2000.

Van den Assum, Laetitia. 2005. 'Towards a UNAIDS Framework Agenda for AIDS and Security'. Report written for UNAIDS (accessed via e-mail to author).

Van der Heijden, Kees. 1996. *Scenarios: The Art of Strategic Conversation*. Chichester: John Wiley and Sons.

Wack, Pierre. 1985a. 'Scenarios: Uncharted Waters Ahead'. *Harvard Business Review*, September–October: 73–89.

———. 1985b. 'Scenarios: Shooting the Rapids'. *Harvard Business Review*, November–December: 139–50.

Conclusion

———•———

Robyn Pharoah

The so-called 'securitisation' of the HIV/AIDS epidemic has both benefited and hindered efforts to combat the virus. On the positive side, the linking of HIV/AIDS to issues of state stability and security by the United Nations (UN) and other agencies has placed what is seen as primarily a developing world problem firmly on the international agenda and helped to marshal the huge – if still insufficient – resources needed to respond to it. On the negative side, advocacy and policy debates have been plagued by 'factoids' – unsubstantiated (and often alarmist) figures and suppositions recycled as fact by a handful of researchers – that have served both to circumvent the critical research and conceptual clarification needed to build effective responses and to raise questions over the strength of the foundation on which they are built.

While there is relatively little empirical data available to illuminate the political and stability effects of the HIV/AIDS epidemic, it is clear that it presents multiple threats to individual well-being in heavily affected countries, such as South Africa. The extraordinarily high levels of adult illness and death heralded by the epidemic clearly undermine the rights of individuals to life and freedom from want and fear, by damaging household and – potentially – national economies, weakening governance structures, hampering service delivery and causing untold anguish and suffering. From this perspective, HIV/AIDS is both a consequence and a symptom of human insecurity. Addressing the epidemic thus requires putting measures in place to enhance and protect well-being at all levels.

A unique epidemic
The HIV/AIDS epidemic is unique in its profile, magnitude and likely duration. By the end of 2003, it had claimed more lives than any other epidemic in recorded

history, with approximately 25 million people worldwide having died of AIDS (UNAIDS 2006). Statistics published by the Joint United Nations Programme on HIV/AIDS (UNAIDS) in mid-2006 suggest that without significant improvements in the availability of treatment, at least 30 million people will die over the next two decades (UNAIDS 2006). Most of these people will be working-age adults in the prime of their lives and while the precise pathways have yet to be understood, the loss of millions of parents, workers, civil servants and politicians will affect societies for generations to come. As several of the preceding authors in this volume have noted, HIV/AIDS is a long-wave event that will play out over decades, perhaps even centuries.

This lengthy time horizon presents the central difficulty in trying to understand and mitigate the long-term effects of the epidemic: it is difficult to conceptualise and respond to threats and challenges that may only be felt years from now and which will undoubtedly last beyond our lifetimes. As Pieter Fourie notes in Chapter 11, the world is only 25 years into an epidemic cycle that may last 50 to 120 years, or more. In this respect, the world is confronting an entirely new phenomenon and it is unlikely that either history or past experience have adequately prepared us for what lies ahead.

The roots of the epidemic

HIV has spread at astonishing speed. As late as 1990, it was estimated that less than 1 per cent of South Africans were HIV-positive. By mid-2006, UNAIDS estimated that about 19 per cent of South Africans – between 4.9 and 6.1 million people – were living with the virus (UNAIDS 2006, 6). Low diagnosis levels, under-reporting and crude estimation tools may have led analysts to underestimate the extent of the early epidemic, particularly in rural areas. However, such figures still point to an extremely steep increase in infection levels over the past seventeen years. There are now more people living with HIV in South Africa than anywhere else in the world.

The factors fuelling the epidemic are varied and complex, but involve features of South Africa's colonial past and apartheid, including impoverishment and disenfranchisement, rapid and disorderly urbanisation and migration. Two factors stand out: large-scale population movements and the violence and social dislocation of the apartheid and post-apartheid period. As Shula Marks argues in Chapter 2, the large-scale movement of people – from the oscillating migration of male labourers from the countryside to the mines, to the more recent flow of poor men and women to urban areas in search of opportunities and the displacements caused by the political unrest of the early 1990s – have all served not only to increase the size of people's sexual networks, but also to spread HIV/AIDS and other infections around the country. This mobility, combined with the violence and political tensions of the late 1970s–90s also served to fracture relationships, increasing social dislocation and concomitantly, vulnerability to infection. The use of rape to intimidate political opponents, particularly in KwaZulu-Natal, may also have served to spread the virus. Without doubt, high levels of violence against women and children continue to facilitate the spread of the virus, while preventing many from undergoing HIV testing or accessing healthcare.

Multilevel, multilayered impacts

The full effects of the epidemic have yet to be felt, but it is widely agreed that HIV/AIDS will have demographic, social, economic and governance consequences that are likely to reverse the gains in life expectancy, poverty reduction, education and healthcare achieved by South Africa and southern Africa as a whole over the last 50 years. In addition to the obvious increases in illness and death, the epidemic is likely to result in rising levels of poverty and vulnerability and, in the absence of widely accessible treatment, inequality, as those with more resources are more easily able to gain access to life-prolonging medicines. Rising levels of illness and death may also increase the cost of doing business, decrease investment and consumption, and reduce the reach, responsiveness and resilience of public institutions, with implications for economic growth and service delivery. Some have speculated that growing poverty and inequality and damage to the credibility and operational effectiveness of government institutions may undermine democracy and even exacerbate or provoke social volatility, political polarisation and conflict.

As is clear from the chapters in this volume, South Africa is already feeling many of these effects. Death rates in the 25–55 age group – which should have the lowest mortality rate – have risen steadily over the last decade, as have infant and child mortality rates. Growing numbers of children are being orphaned. It is estimated that as many as half of all orphans under the age of eighteen have lost parents to HIV/AIDS and it is expected that a vast majority of children will be orphaned by 2015. There is also abundant evidence that the wealth and assets of affected households are being reduced, families are being broken up, traditional coping mechanisms strained and livelihoods threatened. The data wear thin at community and national level, but studies suggest that economic productivity may be declining in heavily affected countries, including South Africa, and that the epidemic may be exacerbating staff and resource shortages in some government departments. Karl Peltzer's findings in Chapter 5 that approximately one in ten of South Africa's existing and student teachers are HIV-positive, for instance, suggest that without treatment, the already overstretched education sector faces considerable losses of expertise and experience over the next decade. Unless this issue is addressed, these losses could impede the South African government's efforts to provide high-quality education to all children. Furthermore, as Razaan Bailey argues in Chapter 8, high HIV prevalence in prison populations may also further strain the already overstretched Department of Correctional Services, as it must care for and treat growing numbers of HIV-positive inmates.

There is, however, little evidence showing if and how the epidemic will impact on traditional security concerns. The information that is available suggests that many early analyses may have overdramatised the implications of the epidemic for stability and security in South Africa. Claims that the disproportionately high levels of infection in the military could leave South Africa unable to defend itself are increasingly being questioned. Rather than being a high-risk population, research conducted by the South African National Defence Force (SANDF) suggests that prevalence rates – at 23 per cent – are on a par with those in the civilian population and some analysts argue that the highly regimented military environment may enable more effective prevention and mitigation strategies. More importantly, although the SANDF has identified HIV/AIDS as a threat to its combat readiness, it is putting in place mechanisms to diagnose, treat and support HIV-positive personnel and their families and there is little reason to believe that the epidemic will weaken the institution sufficiently to compromise national security – or for that matter, that significant military threats to South Africa exist. HIV/AIDS nevertheless remains an important policy issue. As Angela Ndinga-Muvumba suggests in Chapter 9, the prospect of growing regional co-operation for peacekeeping purposes will require greater attention to prevention, the management of HIV-positive soldiers and mitigating the institutional effects of the epidemic.

In terms of national security and crime in South Africa, the suggestion that growing numbers of impoverished orphans may fuel a wave of crime and violence is being interrogated (see Chapter 7 in this volume). While criminological literature suggests that both demographic change and generally higher levels of poverty and vulnerability can create an environment that is more conducive to crime, there is little evidence to suggest that orphans pose a particular risk to security and stability. The few studies that have examined the psycho-social implications of orphaning show that although orphans often experience increased poverty and a range of other social and emotional losses, they are no more prone to crime or violence than other poor children. They also show that the consequences of orphanhood vary according to a range of characteristics and that children orphaned by AIDS are generally no more disadvantaged than poor children living in comparable circumstances. This has led to calls for a shift away from a myopic focus on children orphaned by AIDS to a broader concern for vulnerable children and suggests that the spotlight must remain on the multiple threats to children's well-being, rather than the tenuous threat posed by orphans to security and stability.

The gendered nature of the epidemic

The spread of HIV also has gendered dimensions. As Shula Marks notes in Chapter 2, it is estimated that women are at least twice as likely as men to contract HIV. This is partly due to physiological differences between the sexes, but also largely due to gendered notions of what it means to be male or female in South Africa. Social, political, sexual and economic factors leave many women financially dependent on men, vulnerable to gender-based violence and often with less control over their sexual lives – although factors such as race, marital status, class, age, geographical location and occupation mediate women's susceptibility to the virus. Traditional male gender roles, on the other hand, have been shown to promote negative attitudes towards condom use, while encouraging the belief that men should be sexually aggressive and dominant. The high levels of sexual violence helping to fuel the epidemic may also be rooted in many men's experience of economic exploitation, subordination and lack of control in society. This contradiction between men's ideal role as breadwinners and authority figures has created a crisis of masculinity, which often sees men venting their frustrations on socially weaker women and children.

Men and women also experience the effects of the epidemic differently. In addition to being more vulnerable to infection, women and girls are primarily responsible for caring for the sick and orphaned, while being least equipped to cope materially with this role. HIV-positive women are also more likely than men to face stigma and discrimination, with women commonly blamed for bringing HIV/AIDS into homes. This frequently results in violence and dispossession, with women often being beaten, killed or cast out of their homes. Under traditional land-tenure arrangements, women who lose their husbands to the virus may also lose their right to land and property, as pointed out by Ruth Hall in Chapter 6. While men generally escape the burden of care and experience lower levels of discrimination, gender roles also compromise men's health and well-being. The data emerging from treatment sites, for instance, suggest that men are less likely to access treatment and if they do, it is typically later in the disease cycle than women, when they are often too ill to benefit from treatment.

Despite this evidence, gender issues have yet to be adequately incorporated into policies seeking to counter HIV/AIDS. Abstinence until marriage, for example, is often promoted as the main way for young women to avoid infection. While abstinence is an important prevention strategy, such an approach ignores the fact that many women are unable to abstain for complex social reasons often beyond their control. As observed by Dean Peacock, Thokozile Budaza and Alan Greig in Chapter 4, effective strategies for addressing HIV/AIDS need to involve both men and women and create opportunities for both groups to examine and understand how gender roles interact with the epidemic.

The need for innovative responses

Responding effectively to the implications of HIV/AIDS will also require innovative, locally appropriate interventions. The focus in the first 25 years of the epidemic has been on preventing and treating the virus, but as important as such measures are, the contributions to this volume suggest that they will only partly address the challenges posed by the epidemic. Measures aimed at preventing new infections more effectively and managing those that have already occurred will need to be accompanied by strategies for addressing the human and financial costs of HIV/AIDS in the development and governance sectors in Africa. Decision-makers and practitioners will also need to explore and define new roles and responsibilities for governments, business and civil society, as well as new pathways for collaboration between these actors. Strategies will need to be informed by African-focused research and adopt African solutions that address the realities and challenges faced on the continent. They will also need to be accompanied by appropriate resources and capacity-building efforts.

This is not a simple undertaking. As Alan Whiteside notes in Chapter 10, it is difficult to appreciate the seriousness and implications of a long-wave event such as the HIV/AIDS epidemic. It takes time before there are sufficient deaths for the virus to become visible. Even then, the deaths are distributed widely and, given the stigma associated with HIV/AIDS, remain largely invisible. This invisibility makes it hard to convince key actors of the need to prioritise the effects of the epidemic and mount pre-emptive responses. The likely duration of the epidemic also presents difficulties for programme- and policy-designers. The long-term implications of the epidemic may be far from clear, while actions taken for the ostensible good of sufferers can have long-term consequences that exacerbate the spread and effects of the epidemic. As already mentioned, strategies that make women and girls primarily responsible for preventing infection, for example, may exacerbate the gender-blaming that characterises the HIV/AIDS epidemic in South Africa. Similarly, development projects that facilitate movement and create pockets of wealth in generally impoverished settings may also facilitate the transmission of the virus.

In the context of the epidemic, the South African government's 'business as usual' is simply not an option. Decisive and sustained action is required to maintain and protect the well-being of all South Africans and to avert the worst effects of the epidemic. Strategies need to be instituted urgently to prevent, treat and manage the effects of the virus. Everyone has a role to play and both HIV/AIDS and gender concerns must be mainstreamed into the activities of the public, private and non-governmental sectors. Most importantly, strategies aimed at addressing the virus must complement and feed into activities aimed at maintaining and improving human security in South Africa and the rest of southern Africa. The HIV/AIDS epidemic is fuelled by underdevelopment, while poverty, socio-economic inequality and poor service delivery exacerbate the impact of the virus on those infected and affected by it. It is thus vital that effective mitigation strategies form part of a developmental approach that addresses the underlying vulnerabilities that both drive and worsen the effects of the epidemic.

The transformative potential of the epidemic

Not all the consequences of the HIV/AIDS epidemic are negative. In as much as the epidemic presents challenges to human security in South Africa, it also presents opportunities for positive transformation. In Chapter 6, Ruth Hall describes AIDS-induced changes in traditional land allocation practices that may provide greater security to women and children affected by the epidemic. Edwin Cameron and Marlise Richter argue in Chapter 3 that the epidemic can serve to enhance democratic and human rights principles. They also suggest that agitation by the Treatment Action Campaign (TAC) has not only helped secure the roll-out of antiretroviral (ARV) drugs in South Africa in 2003, but has also transformed HIV/AIDS into a political issue. The epidemic has provided a window on the larger violation of the rights of poor South Africans to health and dignity and enabled political engagement aimed at enhancing democratic and human rights principles in South Africa. In their discussion of the TAC's efforts to address gender-based violence in Chapter 4, Dean Peacock, Thokozile Budaza and Alan Greig demonstrate how activists' efforts to obtain justice for victims of violence have not only made them more aware of the gender dynamics fuelling the epidemic, but have also provided a platform for challenging these dynamics in the communities in which they work. Finally, Angela Ndinga-Muvumba shows in Chapter 9 how the HIV/AIDS epidemic is forcing the South African military to examine questions concerning the rights of soldiers, the role of military medicine and the relationship between militaries and civilian populations.

Creative solutions are being put in place

It is also clear that while many governments and regional and international organisations have been slow to appreciate and respond to the multiple threats posed by the epidemic, creative responses have been developed and applied. The SANDF, for example, has developed an HIV/AIDS intervention strategy with wide-ranging programmatic reach. Under the direction and management of the South African Military Health Services (SAMHS), the South African military has launched an HIV/AIDS education and prevention programme, as well as a clinical research initiative aimed at minimising the spread of the epidemic and improving the management of HIV-positive personnel and their families. The clinical research programme is novel in that it seeks to generate new, context-appropriate knowledge about the challenges of administering ARVs, as well as the utility of African herbs and non-traditional medicines in managing the virus.

Building a community of practice

While there is a need for a great deal more research into the implications of the HIV/AIDS epidemic, particularly the consequences of high HIV prevalence for communities, governance and more traditional security concerns, it is clear that the epidemic constitutes a significant threat to society and human security in South Africa. HIV/AIDS will cause major social changes in South Africa and will alter the face of communities and societies in ways that are still hard to comprehend. The epidemic is, and will continue to be, a significant policy issue, requiring urgent action on the part of governments, the private sector, civil society and individuals. In responding to the epidemic, practitioners, policy-makers and the research community in South Africa will need to think creatively and explore innovative ways of both responding to the epidemic and measuring its effects. The prospect of such change presents an opportunity to address the vulnerabilities and inequalities that fuel the epidemic and to pursue meaningful improvements to human security in South Africa. The implications of the epidemic could be devastating, but with decisive, forward-thinking approaches, HIV/AIDS also presents an unprecedented window of opportunity for creating a better life for all of South Africa's 47 million people.

Reference
UNAIDS (Joint United Nations Programme on HIV/AIDS). 2006. 'Report on the Global AIDS Epidemic'. UNAIDS/06.20E.

Contributors

———— • ————

Razaan Bailey is the project manager of mediation and training services at the Centre for Conflict Resolution (CCR) in Cape Town. She has been working with CCR's Prisons Transformations Project since 2004.

Thokozile Budaza is a gender and HIV/AIDS activist based in Johannesburg. She is a programme officer at the Open Society Institute of Southern Africa.

Edwin Cameron is a Justice of the Supreme Court of Appeal of South Africa. He is the author of *Witness to AIDS* (2005).

Pieter Fourie is the Chair of the Department of Politics at the University of Johannesburg. He is the author of *The Political Management of HIV and AIDS in South Africa: One Burden Too Many?* (2006).

Alan Greig is an independent consultant. He is a writer, trainer and film-maker working on gender, violence and social justice issues, most recently supporting and documenting work with men on masculinity, violence and HIV/AIDS.

Ruth Hall is a researcher at the Programme for Land and Agrarian Studies (PLAAS) at the University of the Western Cape. She is co-editor of *The Land Question in South Africa* (2007).

Shula Marks is Emeritus Professor of History at the School of Oriental and African Studies at the University of London. She is the author of numerous articles and books on a wide variety of subjects, in particular, pertaining to social conditions in South Africa.

Angela Ndinga-Muvumba was the head of the project on HIV/AIDS and security issues at CCR between 2005 and 2008 and is now manager of knowledge production at the African Centre for the Constructive Resolution of Disputes (ACCORD). She is co-editor of *The African Union and Its Institutions* (2008).

Dean Peacock is co-founder and co-director of the Sonke Gender Justice Project. From 2001–05, he was the South Africa programme director for EngenderHealth and assisted many organisations with the implementation of the Men as Partners (MAP) programme, and with the establishment of the National Gender Machinery Working Group on Men and Gender Equality.

Karl Peltzer is the director of the research programme on social aspects of HIV/AIDS and health at the Human Sciences Research Council (HSRC) and is the author of numerous publications.

Robyn Pharoah is an independent consultant based in Cape Town. She was previously a researcher at the Institute for Security Studies (ISS). She is the editor of the ISS monograph *A Generation at Risk? HIV/AIDS, Vulnerable Children and Security in Southern Africa* (2004).

Nana Poku is the John Ferguson Professor of African Studies at the University of Bradford. He was previously director of research for the United Nations Commission on HIV/AIDS and Governance in Africa (UNCHGA) and is the author of *AIDS in Africa: How the Poor are Dying* (2006) and co-editor of *AIDS and Governance* (2007).

Marlise Richter is a researcher at the Reproductive Health and HIV Research Unit (RHRU) of the University of the Witwatersrand. She was previously a researcher at the AIDS Law Project (ALP).

Bjorg Sandkjaer is a programme communications officer at GAVI (Global Alliance for Vaccines and Immunisation). Between 2003 and 2006 she served as an associate demographer for UNCHGA. She is co-editor of *AIDS and Governance* (2007).

Alan Whiteside is the director of the Health Economics and HIV/AIDS Research Division (HEARD) of the University of KwaZulu-Natal and a Professor at the university. He has written widely on HIV/AIDS, most recently *HIV/AIDS: A Very Short Introduction* (2008).

Index

— • —

Note: Page numbers referring to tables and figures are in italics.